Pulmonary Disorders
of the Elderly

Pulmonary Disorders
of the Elderly

*Diagnosis, Prevention,
and Treatment*

EDITORS

Thomas L. Petty, MD, MACP
James S. Seebass, DO, FACOI

American College of Physicians   Philadelphia

Director, Editorial Production: Linda Drumheller
Associate Publisher and Manager, Books Publishing: Tom Hartman
Production Supervisor: Allan S. Kleinberg
Senior Production Editor: Karen C. Nolan
Publishing Coordinator: Angela Gabella
Cover and Interior Design: Kate Nichols
Index: Nelle Garrecht

Printed in the United States of America
Printed by McNaughton & Gunn
Composition by Scribe, Inc. (www.scribenet.com)

ISBN: 1-930513-84-4

The authors and publisher have exerted every effort to ensure that the drug selection and dosages set forth in this book are in accordance with current recommendations and practice at the time of publication. In view of ongoing research, occasional changes in government regulations, and the constant flow of information relating to drug therapy and drug reactions, the reader is urged to check the package insert for each drug for any change in indications and dosage and for additional warnings and precautions. This care is particularly important when the recommended agent is a new or infrequently used drug.

07 08 09 10 11 / 10 9 8 7 6 5 4 3 2 1

Contributors

J. Kern Buckner, MD
South Denver Cardiology Associates
Littleton, Colorado

J. Roy Duke, Jr., MD
Department of Veterans Affairs
West Palm Beach, Florida

James T. Good, Jr., MD
Professor of Medicine
National Jewish Medical and
  Research Center
Denver, Colorado

Leonard D. Hudson, MD, FACP
Professor of Medicine
University of Washington
Seattle, Washington

Thomas M. Hyers, MD, FACP
CARE Clinical Research
St. Louis, Missouri

Michael D. Iseman, MD, FACP
Professor of Medicine
National Jewish Medical and
  Research Center
Denver, Colorado

*Thomas L. Petty, MD, MACP
Professor of Medicine
University of Colorado Health
  Sciences Center
Denver, Colorado

*James S. Seebass, DO, FACOI
Tulsa Health Department
Past Professor and Chair
Department of Medicine
Oklahoma State University Health
  Science Center
Tulsa, Oklahoma

Allan B. Wicks, MD
South Denver Pulmonary Associates
Englewood, Colorado

*Co-Editor

v

Acknowledgments

The authors express their appreciation to Mrs. Kay Bowen for manuscript preparation, to Louise M. Nett for assistance, and to Mrs. Diane Seebass for copy editing. Special appreciation is expressed to Dr. Steven Weinberger for his helpful assistance with the final manuscript.

Contents

Preface

I n 2003, 11% of the United States population was 65 years of age or older. By 2015, that percentage will rise to 14%. In 2003, 34 million persons in the United States were older than 65 years; this number will almost double to 62 million by 2025! Persons over the age of 85 are currently the most rapidly growing segment of our society.

Pulmonary problems increase in frequency with age. Thus the number of persons with respiratory problems and associated comorbidities will increase over the next decades and become an even greater challenge to physicians and other health care providers.

Perhaps the most difficult task is to define the term *elderly*. The sole use of "age" will of necessity exclude "younger" individuals who by physiological criteria are "elderly." In the United States, the minimum age for eligibility for Medicare (65 years) is frequently used to define the minimum age for "elderly," although many of these individuals retain great fitness and excellent physiological profiles. *Pulmonary Disorders of the Elderly: Diagnosis, Prevention, and Treatment* focuses on individuals 65 years and older who have respiratory impairment that negatively affects their quality of life.

Almost no one reaches the age of 65 without some disease or associated illnesses. As respiratory problems become a major cause of morbidity and mortality in the aged, so do comorbidities. Also, pharmacological side effects and drug interactions from therapies must be constantly considered as an integral part of comprehensive management. Acute and chronic pulmonary problems, taken together, threaten the life and happiness of elderly patients more than diseases involving any other organ system. Indeed, pneumonia is the third most common cause of death in the elderly, affecting over one million Americans each year, often at the end of life. A growing number of viral infections can be particularly lethal for older people.

The comorbidities of age are a major associated burden on patients with respiratory disorders. In addition, many common acute and chronic pulmonary problems are often misdiagnosed or overlooked in the elderly. Fortunately, there is an increasing array of preventive and therapeutic agents that deal effectively with most of the respiratory disorders found in the older population.

The authors have collective experience in the treatment of pulmonary and cardiac disorders of over 250 years. We are practitioners and teachers. As a group, we are responsible for the contents of this volume. We offer health care providers both established therapies and new approaches to help them diagnose, treat, and prevent respiratory disorders of the elderly. We trust that *Pulmonary Disorders of the Elderly* will become useful in your practice and remain a key reference in your library.

The Authors

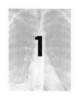

1   The Aging Lung

L ung structure and function change with aging. The maximum number of alveoli is reached at about 10-12 years of age, and maximal function is achieved in young adulthood, generally in the early 20s. After a relatively short plateau in lung function, progressive decline occurs over the remainder of life. Despite this gradual decline, the respiratory system is able to maintain adequate gas exchange throughout the entire lifespan, unless affected by disease. The structural changes in the lung and the resulting lung functional changes that occur with aging are reviewed here.

Structural Changes

The major structural changes occurring in the lung are: 1) changes in the lung parenchyma that decrease elastic recoil; 2) stiffening of the chest wall; and 3) associated changes in respiratory muscle function. Elastic recoil decreases as part of the normal aging process. The total lung content of collagen and elastin is unchanged, and qualitative changes in these lung constituents appear to explain the loss of elastic recoil. Collagen cross-linking changes with age, and elastic fibers degenerate and lose their elasticity. Both of these changes result in a net loss of elastic recoil and enlargement of alveolar ducts and alveoli. These changes are histologically different from those of emphysema in that there is no destruction of the alveolar walls. However, they result in similar changes in lung compliance. These changes have been inappropriately called "senile emphysema."

Chest wall compliance decreases progressively with age. This stiffening is presumably related to calcification of costal cartilage and the articulations between the ribs and the vertebrae, in addition to narrowing of intervertebral disc spaces. Age-related osteoporosis can result in vertebral wedge (partial) or crush (complete) fractures with accompanying dorsal kyphosis and increased anteroposterior (AP) chest diameter (barrel chest). These osteoporosis-related changes occur twice as commonly in females as in males. In one study, wedge vertebral fractures were found in 60% of females aged 75 years and older and more than 7% of females had vertebral crush fractures. These modifications of the chest wall result in stiffening, affecting the curvature of the diaphragm and decreasing its ability to generate forces.

Respiratory muscle function is also impaired with increasing age. There are several reasons for this. The increase in functional residual capacity (end-expiratory resting lung volume) due to the loss of elastic recoil and the development of kyphosis and increased AP diameter described above place the chest wall muscles and the diaphragm in a less advantageous position to generate forces than in younger individuals without these changes.

Age-associated changes in peripheral skeletal muscles have been well studied and include a decrease in the number of muscle fibers, especially "fast twitch" fibers, changes in neuromuscular junctions, and loss of peripheral motor neurons. At the cellular level, impairment of calcium pumps involved in cytoplasmic reticulum and uncoupling of ATP hydrolysis and calcium transport can contribute to a reduction in contraction velocity. A decreased synthesis of muscle myosin and a decrease in mitochondrial respiratory chain function also can contribute to reduced skeletal muscle performance. It is very likely that these same changes occur in respiratory skeletal muscles and affect their function. Respiratory muscle function is related to nutritional status, which is often suboptimal in the elderly. Respiratory muscle function is also dependent on energy availability, which may be limited by comorbid diseases. For example, it has been demonstrated that patients with chronic congestive heart failure have a decrease in respiratory muscle strength.

Lung Functional Changes

Total lung capacity (TLC) does not change significantly throughout life. The decreased elastic recoil of the lungs that occurs with increasing age is counterbalanced by an increasing elastic load due to the stiffness of the chest wall. However, there are significant changes within the volumes, which make up the total lung capacity. These changes are primarily an increase in residual volume (RV) and functional residual capacity (FRC), with a corresponding decrease in vital capacity (VC) (Figure 1-1). The air trapping that increases the RV and FRC is a result of age-related decreased elastic recoil of the lung tissue, premature closure of small airways, and increased stiffness of the chest wall. Therefore, older individuals breathe at higher lung volumes than younger subjects due to the shape of the static pressure-volume curve of the respiratory system. The increase in FRC places an added burden on the respiratory muscles and increases breathing-related energy expenditure in older, compared with younger, individuals. It is estimated that a 60-year-old man has a 20% increase in breathing-related energy expenditure compared with a 20-year-old man.

The closing volume (CV), the lung volume at which dependent small airways begin to close during exhalation, also increases with age. This premature airway closure is presumably related to the changes in the elastic fiber makeup, resulting in poor support or tethering around the terminal airways. This can have a significant effect on gas exchange because airway closure can begin to occur during a normal tidal breath, resulting in a ventilation/perfusion mismatch. This phenomenon is the major explanation for the age-related decrease in oxygenation.

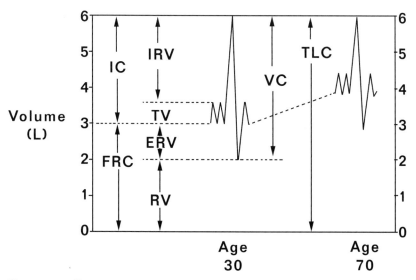

Figure 1-1 Changes in spirogram with subdivision of lung volumes occurring with aging. TLC = total lung capacity; VC = vital capacity; IC = inspiratory capacity; FRC = functional residual capacity; IRV = inspiratory reserve volume; TV = tidal volume; ERV = expiratory reserve volume; RV = residual volume. TLC remains unchanged with increasing age; FRC and RV increase, and VC decreases. Also (not shown), elastic recoil decreases, resulting in a decrease in forced expiratory flow rates.

Forced expiratory volume in 1 second (FEV_1) and forced vital capacity (FVC) begin to diminish in the mid-20s. The annual decrease in FEV_1 is approximately 20 mL/year in subjects up to age 40 and is approximately double that once an individual's age is greater than 65. The decrease in FEV_1 is slightly greater than the decrease in FVC, particularly from age 50 to 60 on, resulting in a decrease in the FEV_1/FVC ratio in older individuals.

These normal changes in lung structure and function have modest effects on oxygenation. The alveolar-to-arterial oxygen difference increases with age primarily due to the increased closing volume discussed above, with airway closure in dependent lung units occurring during tidal breathing. However, in individuals who do not have additional lung disease, arterial PaO_2 remains well above that required for nearly complete saturation of the hemoglobin (≥95%) in individuals at sea level.

Carbon monoxide diffusing capacity (DLCO) also decreases with increasing age, usually occurring after age 40. This is due to the structural changes described above and also to an increased heterogeneity of ventilation/perfusion. The decline in the DLCO is probably related to some reduction in the density of capillaries of the lung and pulmonary capillary blood volume.

Regulation of Breathing

Changes in regulation of breathing also occur with increasing age. The responses to hypercapnia and hypoxia are blunted in older individuals, though the underlying mechanisms for this change are not known. This does not affect normal resting minute ventilation, despite the fact that older subjects breathe with smaller tidal volumes and higher respiratory rates than younger subjects. However, these blunted ventilatory responses could have clinically important effects with added breathing loads and under disease conditions.

The prevalence of sleep-disordered breathing is increased in elderly subjects. The repetitive episodes of upper airway obstruction increase with increasing age; additionally, the respiratory effort in response to this obstruction is decreased in the elderly compared with younger people.

Defense Mechanisms

Mucociliary clearance declines in old age, as does lung macrophage function. Cell-mediated immunity also begins to fail. The alveolar macrophage plays an important protective role as a first line of defense. Although not shown to diminish in number with age, multiple medical conditions exist in the elderly that are known to impair macrophage function. The decreased ability to generate a T lymphocyte immune response has been found in the elderly. Polymorphonuclear leukocytes, while normal in number, appear to have a diminished reserve of precursor cells. Defects in chemotaxis, phagocytosis, and bactericidal activity of neutrophils have been noted. Immunosenescence is known to progress with aging, as is shown by the decreased activity of cell-mediated and humoral immunity. These may be reasons for the increased susceptibility of elderly persons to respiratory infections of all causes.

BIBLIOGRAPHY AND SUGGESTED READING

Crapo RO. The aging lung. In: Mahler DA, ed. Pulmonary Disease in the Elderly Patient, vol 63. New York: Marcel Dekker; 1993:1-21. *An authoritative chapter on this subject. Although more than a decade old, most of the information is still relevant.*

Janssens JP, Pache JC, Nicod LP. Physiological changes in respiratory function associated with aging. Eur Respir J. 1999;13:197-205. *An excellent review of the structural and functional changes in the lung with aging. Thorough, yet concise and well-referenced.*

2 Dyspnea and Cough

We have made great strides in pulmonary medicine since the days of "consumption" and "the catarrh." However, with our aging population and advanced diagnostic techniques, we are now seeing an increase in lung disease. It is evident that physicians will be increasingly called upon to evaluate the elderly for a variety of respiratory symptoms. These symptoms carry more significance in the aging population for several reasons. First, the odds of a symptom representing significant disease increase as one ages. Second, older individuals usually recognize their mortality: they have seen friends, co-workers, and family members develop warning symptoms, receive serious diagnoses, and subsequently die. When confronted with symptomatic elderly patients, the physician should be aware of these patients' deep concerns about their complaints.

Three complaints represent the great majority of primary care referrals to the pulmonologist for consultation: dyspnea, cough (especially when chronic), and an abnormal chest x-ray. This chapter addresses dyspnea and the chronic cough.

Dyspnea

Pathophysiology

The physiological mechanisms of dyspnea are multiple and complex. Despite the importance and frequency of the symptoms of dyspnea, our knowledge of the underlying mechanisms is still incomplete. Through a complex interaction involving J stretch fibers in the alveolar interstitium, muscle spindle fibers, the carotid body chemoreceptors, and neural pathways, patients experience the sensation of breathlessness. There are three basic underlying mechanisms of dyspnea:

1) Increased awareness of normal breathing as seen in anxiety and hyperventilation
2) Increased work of breathing due to either airway obstruction or restrictive lung disease with loss of compliance
3) Abnormality of the ventilatory apparatus as seen in neuromuscular disease, obesity, and thoracic cage abnormalities

Full discussion of these mechanisms is beyond the scope of this chapter; readers are referred to an excellent monograph, *Dyspnea: Frontline Cardio-Pulmonary Topics*, for a more extensive review.

Evaluation

The elderly individual undergoes many changes in the respiratory system (see Chapter 1). Some of these changes include a decreased ventilatory response to chemical stimuli, progressive decline in lung function, and a decline in respiratory muscle strength. Such changes, when combined with comorbid disease and physical deconditioning, because of a decreased activity level, are often expressed as "shortness of breath." However, dyspnea should never be attributed to the "normal aging process" without a thorough investigation. It is often a dramatic and frightening experience for the older patient. An initial history and physical examination alone will quite often establish the etiology. When a diagnosis is not established, appropriate testing should be undertaken. This evaluation is most commonly directed at the cardiopulmonary systems because they account for 75% of the causes of dyspnea. If these two systems are eliminated as a cause, physical deconditioning, anemia, and psychogenic factors should be considered.

The history and physical examination can provide many clues in the diagnostic evaluation of dyspnea. Establish whether the dyspnea is of acute onset (24-48 hours). When dyspnea is acute, the differential diagnosis is dramatically reduced, including pulmonary embolism, pneumothorax, acute asthma, congestive heart failure, myocardial infarction, or cardiac tamponade. Studies have shown that the history and physical examination alone establish the diagnosis in 70-80% of the cases of acute-onset dyspnea. The etiology may be multifactorial in up to one-third of these cases.

Chronic dyspnea is commonly encountered in clinical practice and can be caused by any progressive lung disease or cardiac problem. The frequency of both chronic pulmonary diseases and cardiac diseases increases with age. Anemia, deconditioning, and a number of other non-cardiopulmonary conditions can cause or contribute to chronic dyspnea; these factors are more common in the elderly than in younger individuals.

Pertinent questioning can provide valuable information and diagnostic clues to the cause of dyspnea. A history of pre-existing cardiac or lung disease should be sought because dyspnea may represent worsening of the underlying process. Factors such as duration, precipitating events, association with exertion, day or night occurrence, and associated symptoms such as coughing and wheezing may give more insight into the etiology. Other factors to be considered include past and current tobacco use and occupational, environmental, and drug history. Dyspnea with positional characteristics (orthopnea, trepopnea, and platypnea) will suggest specific diagnoses (Table 2-1).

A complete examination for physical findings often leads the physician toward a proper diagnosis and may minimize extensive, expensive, and unnecessary laboratory testing. Following visual inspection of the chest, which can give clues, specific attention should focus on the neck, lungs, and heart. The neck is evaluated specifically for jugular venous distention and cervical and supraclavicular adenopathy. Tactile fremitus is decreased in emphysema and increased with pulmonary consolidation. Parenchymal disease can present with crackles and findings of consolidation. Auscultation of the lungs can demonstrate such evidence of airway disease as wheezing, prolonged expiratory phase, diminished breath sounds, and sonorous rhonchi. Pleural effusion is demonstrated by dullness to percussion with absent breath sounds. Cardiac examination may indicate disease when murmurs, abnormal PMI, arrhythmias, or an extra heart sound is found. Specific findings and associated diagnoses in patients with dyspnea are listed in Table 2-2.

After a thorough history and physical examination, the clinician should be able to determine whether the etiology of the dyspnea is most likely cardiac

Table 2-1 Diagnostic Considerations in Positional Dyspnea

Orthopnea	Dyspnea during reclining, relieved in upright position	Congestive heart failure, COPD, bilateral diaphragm paralysis
Platypnea	Dyspnea in upright position, improved with reclining (associated with orthodeoxia)	Hepatopulmonary syndrome with right-to-left shunt, right-to-left shunt through patent foramen ovale
Trepopnea	Dyspnea in right or left lateral decubitus position	Damaged lung with fibrosis or tumor with affected lung dependent

Table 2-2 Specific Findings and Primary Diagnostic Considerations in Patients with Dyspnea

Specific Physical Findings	Examples of Diagnoses
General Observations	
Obesity	Deconditioning
Clubbing	Interstitial lung disease
	Bronchiectasis
	Neoplasm
	Cystic fibrosis
	Congenital heart disease
Kyphoscoliosis	Restrictive lung disease
Barrel chest	Chronic obstructive pulmonary disease (COPD)
Abnormal breathing	Congestive heart failure (CHF)
	Central nervous system disease
Use of accessory muscles for breathing	Asthma
	COPD
Pallor	Anemia
Edema/ascites	CHF
	Hepatic disease
Cardiovascular Observations	
Elevated jugular venous distension	CHF/pericardial disease/cor pulmonale or hepatojugular reflux
Delayed carotid upstroke	Aortic stenosis (AS)
Parasternal lift	Pulmonary hypertension
Diffuse apical impulse	Left ventricular (LV) enlargement, systolic dysfunction
Sustained apical impulse	LV hypertrophy, diastolic dysfunction
Increased S1	Mitral stenosis
Increased P2	Pulmonary hypertension
Fixed split S2	Atrial septal defect (ASD)
Single S2	AS
S3 gallop	Systolic dysfunction/CHF
S4 gallop	Diastolic dysfunction
Diastolic murmur	Valvular heart disease (pathologic)
Pulsus alternans	LV dysfunction
Pulsus paradoxus	Cardiac tamponade
	Asthma

Continued.

Table 2-2 Specific Findings and Primary Diagnostic Considerations in Patients with Dyspnea *(Continued)*

Specific Physical Findings	Examples of Diagnoses
Pulmonary Observations	
Increased tactile fremitus	Pneumonia (consolidation)
Decreased tactile fremitus	Pleural effusion
	Pneumothorax
Dullness to percussion	Atelectasis
	Pleural effusion
	Pneumonia
Hyperresonance	Emphysema
Bronchial or tubular breath sounds	Pneumonia
Crackles (alveolar disease)	CHF
	Idiopathic pulmonary fibrosis
	Pneumonia
Rhonchi (airway disease)	Bronchitis
	COPD
Egophony	Consolidation

Republished with permission from Petty TL, Smith SC. Dyspnea. Frontline Cardio-Pulmonary Topics. Denver: Snowdrift Pulmonary Conference; 2001:76.

or pulmonary in origin or whether it results from other disease states. Clinical testing should then be directed appropriately. If etiology is still unclear, the standard screening tests should be undertaken. These include spirometry, chest x-ray, oximetry, and electrocardiogram.

Spirometry identifies and quantifies the extent of airway disease or lung restriction. Rarely does a patient with airway disease experience significant dyspnea until the FEV_1 is at or below 50% of predicted. Spirometry should diagnose the majority of patients with COPD and asthma. If the forced vital capacity is reduced and the FEV_1/FVC is normal or is increased above 70%, a restrictive process should be considered and complete lung volumes measured.

The PA and lateral chest radiographs are an essential part of the work-up. Both parenchymal pulmonary disease and cardiac enlargement can be demonstrated. However, significant underlying cardiac and pulmonary disease can be present with a normal chest x-ray.

Oximetry is a valuable, rapid, and widely available non-invasive procedure that has been incorporated in many primary care offices. It is easily performed and accurate in most clinical situations. However, like the EKG and chest x-ray, normal results do not rule out significant disease. If normal initially, oximetry can be repeated with exercise and if found to be abnormal, indicates underlying disease.

Table 2-3 Stepwise Approach to Evaluation of Patient with Chronic Dyspnea

Complexity	Evaluation	Cost*	Risk	Need for Consultation?
All patients with dyspnea	History and physical examination	$	None	No
Diagnosis still not obvious	Spirometry Electrocardiogram (ECG) Chest x-ray (CXR) Oximetry	$ $ $ $	None	No
Diagnosis still not obvious	Arterial blood gases Standard sinus X-rays Full pulmonary function testing Exercise testing Echocardiogram	$ $ $$ $$$ $$$	Minimal	No
Diagnosis still not obvious	Ventilation-perfusion (V/Q) scan	$$	None	No
Diagnosis still not obvious	Chest CT scan Sinus CT scan Stress echo Stress perfusion studies	$$$ or $$$$ (all)	Minimal	Yes
Diagnosis still not obvious	Right and left heart catheterizations	$$$$$	Low	Yes

*These are approximate costs, based on Medicare relative values. Regional and institutional differences can be expected.
$ = $0 to $200; $$ = $201 to $500; $$$ = $501 to $1000; $$$$ = $1001 to $5000; $$$$$ = >$5000.
Republished with permission from Petty TL, Smith SC. Dyspnea. Frontline Cardio-Pulmonary Topics. Denver: Snowdrift Pulmonary Conference; 2001.

The electrocardiogram may give an indication of underlying cardiopulmonary abnormalities when an old myocardial infarction, ischemia, hypertrophy, or arrhythmia is found. These results would necessitate a more extensive evaluation. If the results do not point to a diagnosis, further testing with ABGs, PFTs, exercise testing, echocardiogram, and CT scan may be warranted. Specialized tests and consultations are indicated if an etiology is not found. See Table 2-3.

Cough

Cough is a second symptom commonly encountered in the elderly and is a special concern when it becomes chronic. A 1993 National Ambulatory Medical Care Survey stated that cough was the most common symptom for which adult patients seek medical care in the United States. The complaint of cough, especially chronic cough, may represent as much as 38%

of a pulmonologist's practice, which often includes elderly patients. The importance of knowing how to diagnose and treat cough is further emphasized by the yearly $1 billion in sales of over-the-counter cough suppressants. An etiology of cough should always be sought. However, in one survey 23% of primary care physicians advised their patients to "learn to live" with their cough (Irwin and Madison 2002).

Pathophysiology

The anatomy of a cough involves a complex reflex arc, beginning with the irritation of nerve endings in the ciliated epithelial cells of the respiratory tract. These cough receptor sites are located between the pharynx and the terminal bronchi but have their heaviest concentration where airflow patterns change—in the posterior pharynx and the carina. The sites are superficial and irritated by local infections and mucus movement. They send a signal, usually via the cranial nerves, to the cough center in the upper brain stem and pons, which in turn send the signal to the respiratory muscles to generate an effective cough. In addition, there are non-respiratory cough receptor sites located in the stomach, pericardium, and the tympanic membrane.

Evaluation

In a Consensus Panel Report (Irwin et al 1998) on cough, the expert panel chose to divide cough into acute and chronic, using an arbitrary 3 weeks' duration as the dividing time. However, a later review (Irwin and Madison 2000) added a subacute classification as shown below:

- *Acute*: 3 weeks or less
- *Subacute*: 3 to 8 weeks
- *Chronic*: 8 weeks and greater

This classification is also used in the most recent guidelines developed by the American College of Chest Physicians (Irwin et al 2006).

Acute cough is most commonly viral in origin and is transient. Other common causes of acute cough include bacterial sinusitis, allergic rhinitis, exacerbations of chronic obstructive lung disease, and environmental rhinitis. However, acute cough may represent the initial presenting symptom of more significant underlying disease such as congestive heart failure (CHF), pneumonia, asthma, or pulmonary embolism. The initial history and physical examination in this acute group will most often establish a diagnosis.

Guidelines for therapy of acute cough recommend an approach based on trials of empiric therapy. Antibiotics are not recommended by the American College of Physicians (ACP) for acute cough associated with acute respiratory tract infections.

Subacute cough (3-8 weeks' duration) may often be associated with a prior upper respiratory tract infection. This by itself can lead to postinfectious cough but also may represent the cough of bronchial hyperresponsiveness or post-nasal drip seen after infection. Other causes of subacute cough include bacterial sinusitis, asthma, and the new resurgence of pertussis. Again, as with the acute group, a trial of empiric therapy is recommended if a post-infectious process is suspected. Limited laboratory testing may be indicated when an obvious recent respiratory tract infection is not established. A sinus x-ray series (currently being replaced by sinus CT scans), chest x-ray, and pulmonary function testing may then be indicated in an attempt to identify the etiological basis of the subacute cough.

A patient with a *chronic or "troublesome" cough* has most often been evaluated without receiving a diagnosis prior to being seen by a pulmonologist. (This chapter will not address chronic cough caused by obvious sources such as smoking, lung cancer, or an ACE inhibitor.)

By definition, the chronic cough is seen in a patient who is immuno-competent, has a normal chest x-ray, is a non-smoker with no environmental exposure, and has no obvious explanation for the cough. Chronic cough as defined above may have a major impact on the quality of life of the individual. One study followed patients with cough for an average of 56 months and found that they were more affected by the interference in social interactions than by any physical concern: more than half of them expressed embarrassment because of their cough and believed others thought they had a serious illness.

Successful treatment of this group resulted in dramatic improvement in their quality of life when the cough resolved. The most common reason given for seeking medical care was the need for reassurance that nothing was seriously wrong. When patients with chronic cough are evaluated, the majority have one or more of three etiologies. Seven studies involving 570 patients found that 34% had cough due to post-nasal drainage (now referred to as upper airway cough syndrome), 28% due to asthma, and 18% due to gastroesophageal reflux disease (GERD). A surprising finding was that up to 53% of the time, two of these etiologies were present in chronic cough and 35% of the time all three could be identified (Irwin and Madison 2002). Additional studies have shown that with careful evaluation a cause of chronic cough can be determined in 88-100% of the cases. Treatment was successful 84-98% of the time.

The history and physical examination are valuable tools in evaluating chronic cough. A careful history can often narrow the list of etiologies. The character, timing, and quality of the cough have classically been taught to be valuable, but this has not been proven. More important is questioning for symptoms related to the three most common causes. Even then, one study showed significant overlap of symptoms in GERD, asthma, and post-nasal drainage. For example, 28% of patients diagnosed as asthmatic had no wheezing and only a cough, and 43% of patients diagnosed with GERD had no heartburn or dyspepsia.

The physical exam can give a strong indication that post-nasal drainage is present when oropharyngeal cobblestoning, streaking, and drainage are seen along with allergic nasal findings. In asthma, a prolonged expiratory phase may be found with a wheeze during forced vital capacity maneuvers.

An extensive laboratory and radiographic evaluation is rarely rewarding. A normal chest x-ray makes the three most common culprits more likely. Simple spirometry can help eliminate or establish asthma or COPD as the problem. CT scanning, bronchoscopy, and other sophisticated testing seldom reveal the source of the cough at first. CT can reveal a carcinoma. A lung cancer should always be suspected in current or former elderly smokers who have a cough that persists beyond 3 months, failing empiric therapy. The current approach to treatment is to try therapeutic modalities directed at the three most common causes to see if the cough resolves. A trial of antihistamine-decongestant combination for post-nasal drip is the first step in empiric therapy. If this is not effective, an inhaled beta-agonist is often used to treat cough-variant asthma, which is then followed, if necessary, by treatment for GERD. If none of these treatments is effective, further evaluation may be warranted.

Post-nasal drainage represents the most common cause of chronic cough. This has been most recently renamed "upper airway cough syndrome" by a Committee of the American College of Chest Physicians in 2006 (Irwin et al 2006). Clinically, the patients complain of tickling in the throat and are continually trying to clear the sensation by coughing. Their exams demonstrate cobblestoning, streaking, and mucus drainage in the oropharynx. The oropharynx is richly innervated with superficial cough receptors, and irritation from post-nasal drainage results in cough. The drainage may be due to chronic sinusitis or allergic or non-allergic rhinitis. Often lozenges containing topical anesthetics or aerosolized lidocaine will give temporary relief by anesthetizing the cough receptors in the oropharynx. This treatment may help to establish the diagnosis. The specific therapeutic approach to chronic sinusitis and either allergic or non-allergic rhinitis differs, but one common modality is the use of first-generation antihistamines. They are more effective drying agents than the currently popular non-sedating antihistamines, which do not have significant anticholinergic actions, in contrast to diphenhydramine (Benadryl) and chlorpheniramine (Chlor-Trimeton). Long-term antibiotics and decongestants may be needed for chronic bacterial rhinosinusitis, and ipratropium bromide can be used for non-allergic rhinitis, in addition to a first-generation antihistamine. Saline nasal washes often have a dramatic impact on the resolution of nasal drainage.

Cough-variant asthma has long been recognized as an etiology for chronic cough. Although reports vary as to its prevalence, cough may be the sole manifestation in up to half the cases of asthma (Irwin and Madison 2002). There is nothing distinctive about this cough. A family history of asthma, seasonal occurrence, or a history suggesting a trigger mechanism such as exercise or strong odors may give the physician a clue. Simple office spirometry is the first test to be performed with chronic cough, and this may establish the diagnosis. If doubt remains, an empiric trial of inhaled beta-agonists and steroids can be tried. If a question remains, then a methacholine challenge, although not uniformly available, can be considered as a next step.

GERD is increasingly being recognized as a common etiology of chronic cough. When GERD symptoms are present, the diagnosis is clear. However, at least half of the patients demonstrated to have GERD have no symptoms. Currently a clinical trial of therapy, including an anti-reflux diet, elevation of the head of the patient's bed, acid suppression, and prokinetic agents, is recommended. If the patient is symptomatic, the symptoms of GERD rapidly improve, but the cough may persist for up to 6 months after institution of therapy. If after 3 months there is no improvement, a 24-hour esophageal pH monitor may be considered; however, this is expensive, not widely available, and has a specificity of only 66% in identifying reflux.

Other causes of chronic cough are significantly less common but must be kept in mind. These include chronic suppurative bronchitis, eosinophilic bronchitis (characterized by chronic cough and sputum eosinophilia), pertussis ("the cough of 100 days"), and bronchiectasis.

In a recent monograph presenting the American College of Chest Physicians Evidence-Based Clinical Practice Guidelines on the Diagnosis and Management of Cough, an extensive review of other less common etiologies of cough is presented to include non-bronchiectatic suppurative airway disease, aspiration, environmental and occupational etiologies, and cough in the dialysis patient. This thorough and extensive review of the subject provides an outstanding treatise on acute, subacute, and chronic cough (Irwin et al 2006).

Summary

Dyspnea and chronic cough represent significant complaints from the elderly. Approximately 75% of dyspnea is cardiac or pulmonary in origin, and excellent tests exist to identify the problem. Chronic cough with its strict definition most commonly represents one or more of three problems: GERD, post nasal drainage (upper airway cough syndrome), and asthma.

Chest x-rays and pulmonary function tests are appropriately done in patients with chronic dyspnea and cough. If negative, more extensive evaluations, such as sinus films and studies to confirm GERD, are appropriate, as is additional consultation.

BIBLIOGRAPHY AND SUGGESTED READING

Dyspnea: Mechanisms, Assessment, and Management, A Consensus Statement. Am J Respir Crit Care Med. 1999;159:321-40. *The most recent consensus statement on the pathophysiology, assessment, and treatment of dyspnea.*

Gonzales R, Bartlett JG, Besser RE, et al. Principles of appropriate antibiotic use for treatment of uncomplicated acute bronchitis: background. Ann Emerg Med. 2001;37:720-7.

Harding S, Richter J. The role of gastroesophageal reflux in chronic cough on quality of life. Arch Intern Med. 1998;158. *Review of GERD's role in chronic cough.*

Irwin RS, Madison JM. The diagnosis and treatment of cough. N Engl J Med. 2000;343:1715-21. *A general review of cough and treatment.*

Irwin RS, Madison JM. The persistently troublesome cough. Am J Respir Crit Care Med. 2002;165:1469-74. *An outstanding review of cough and treatment.*

Irwin RS, Baumann MH, Bolser DC, et al. Diagnosis and Management of Cough. Executive Summary: ACCP Evidence-Based Clinical Practice Guidelines. Chest. 2006;129:1-292 (Supplement). *Outstanding and most recent treatise on the subject of cough.*

Irwin RS, Boulet LP, Cloutier MM, et al. Managing cough as a defense mechanism and as a symptom. A consensus panel report of the American College of Chest Physicians. Chest. 1998;114:133S-181S.

Petty TL, Smith SC. Dyspnea. Frontline Cardio-Pulmonary Topics. Denver: Snowdrift Pulmonary Conference; 2001. *A short but complete description of the diagnosis and treatment of dyspnea.*

Morgan WC, Hodge HL. Diagnostic evaluation of dyspnea. Am Fam Phys. 1998;67:233-8. *A concise article on evaluation of dyspnea.*

Silverstri GA, Mahler DA. Evaluation of dyspnea in the elderly patient. Clin Chest Med. 1993;14:393-404. *An entire issue devoted to pulmonary disease in the elderly. The article on dyspnea is an excellent overview.*

3 Influenza and Other Viral Infections

Viruses were first recognized as infectious agents of tobacco in 1892. They were found to be so small that they could pass through filters fine enough to capture all known (bacterial) pathogens. We know now that there are extraordinary arrays of viruses that incorporate diverse structural and functional features, and these microorganisms produce a continually expanding spectrum of human diseases. Contemporary classifications of viruses are based on:

1. Type and structure of nucleic acid (e.g., RNA or DNA)
2. Replication strategy
3. Morphologic symmetry of the viral capsid (either helical or icosahedral [20 equilateral triangles on the surface])
4. Presence or absence of a lipid envelope

Viral nucleic acids are packaged by a protein coat called a *capsid,* composed of individual subunits called *capsomeres*, which contain minimal genetic information for transcription and replication. All viruses must capture the sophisticated cellular processes of host cells for reproduction. To accomplish this essential function, the viruses may act as a "delivery system" (which protects against environmental degradation and promotes attachment to the target host cell) and a "payload" (the genome and enzymes necessary to initiate replication). Viruses with lipid envelopes generally resist environmental degradation and are more prone to airborne transmission.

Aging patients may be less likely to be infected during epidemics because they are less mobile and often avoid crowds and major social events. Once infected, however, the older patient has reduced immunological responses to the infecting agent and thus a worse prognosis than in younger patients.

Although a plethora of viruses have been associated with respiratory infections, the vast majority of the latter are caused by a limited number of species. The predominant viral respiratory pathogens include the influenza, corona, adeno, rhino, parainfluenza, and respiratory syncytial viruses. Some, such as the common cold, may be caused by numerous viruses, whereas others, such as influenza and severe acute respiratory syndrome (SARS) are fairly restrictive within a particular species.

Although there may be considerable overlap, it is clinically useful to characterize infections as upper or lower respiratory tract syndromes (Table 3-1). In many cases, a viral infection may, in fact, progress from one syndrome to several others: coryza ("cold") to pharyngitis, to laryngitis, to bronchitis, and even on to pneumonia. Further complicating matters, an illness of viral origin may be complicated by bacterial superinfection, particularly in the elderly. However, for patients with an illness that clearly fits into a syndromic classification, reasonable inferences may be made regarding the etiologic agent, treatment, and prognosis.

Influenza

Three influenzae genera of importance in human disease are labeled A, B, and C. The A viruses are the most consistent and important of the genera, although there is enough B disease that vaccines include these strains in addition to the A strains. The strains of A that circulate are identified by variants of the major surface antigens, hemagglutinin (HA) and neuraminidase (NA); the current nomenclature also includes the host of origin (e.g., avian or swine), the geographic site of first isolation (e.g., Hong Kong), the strain number, and the year of initial identification. These viruses have often been of the H_3/N_2 genotype.

Generally, the A strains drift antigenically from year to year. However, shifts have occurred in which significantly altered strains appear that involve such a major deviation in antigenicity and virulence that major, lethal pandemics occur. Examples include the Spanish flu pandemic of 1918-19 that took over 40 million lives (the most lethal epidemic ever recorded, including HIV), the Asian flu of 1957, and the Hong Kong flu of 1968.

Recently the so-called avian or bird flu has caused epidemics in chickens in Asia and the Middle East. This virus is H_5N_1. Thus far no human-to-human transfer has been documented; however, as of late summer 2006, approximately 180 deaths, including young children, have occurred worldwide.

Table 3-1 Viral Respiratory Syndromes in the Elderly

Syndrome	Features	Typical Viral Pathogens
Upper Respiratory Infection (URI)		
Common cold	• Coryza with nasal congestion, sneezing, watery discharge, sore throat, cough (nonproductive), +/- low-grade fever and malaise • Typically in colder months (school clustering, time indoors) • Peak incidence: 6 to 8 colds per 1000 persons per day	• Rhinovirus • Coronavirus • Parainfluenza virus • Respiratory syncytial virus • Adenovirus
Pharyngitis	• Most commonly an element of the common cold • Also seen with acute HIV infection or infectious mononucleosis • Prominent element of influenza • Clinically, hard to distinguish from streptococcal pharyngitis	• As above (Common cold) plus coxsackievirus A, Epstein-Barr virus, and HIV-1 virus
Acute laryngitis	• Recent onset of hoarseness or rough voice with deepened pitch • May progress to aphonia	• As above (Common cold); the primary etiologic agent may vary by time and location
Acute sinusitis	• Almost universally follows/is related to a viral URI • Acute symptoms overlap the common cold: sneezing, nasal discharge, nasal obstruction, facial pressure, headache • Original discharge is clear, mucoid, and profuse; may evolve to purulence and discoloration	• As above (Common cold); none of the usual signs/symptoms allow the clinician to distinguish viral from bacterial from mixed etiology
Lower Respiratory Infection (LRI)		
Acute bronchitis	• Cough is the sentinel feature; low-grade fever is common • Increasing frequency and severity of cough • Initially dry, then productive of scanty mucoid secretions; if protracted may yield grossly purulent phlegm • Burning substernal pain suggests severe tracheitis	• Influenza virus • Adenovirus • Rhinovirus • Coronavirus
Pneumonia	• Cough is universal • Fever in the great majority • Dyspnea and tachypnea in nearly all cases • Pleurisy (with/without friction rubs) is rare but more prominent with coxsackievirus and adenovirus pneumonia	• Influenza virus • Adenovirus • Coronavirus (SARS) • Coxsackievirus A

Diagnosis

The clinical manifestations of influenza are well known to physicians: the abrupt onset of a febrile illness associated with headache; chills without rigors; and dry cough progressing to disabling myalgias, malaise, and lassitude. Sore throat, nasal congestion and conjunctival inflammation are common. The acute illness typically lasts 4-6 days, but patients commonly have protracted (10-21 days) cough, respiratory compromise, and debilitating fatigue.

Clinical or radiographic pneumonia due to the influenza virus is found among "normal" hosts and may result in life-threatening hemorrhagic viral pneumonitis. This was a common cause of death in the 1918–19 epidemic. However, secondary bacterial infections of the lower airways may evolve more commonly, particularly in the elderly, due presumably to damage and dysfunction of the ciliated epithelium of the airways (Sethi 2002). Clues to secondary pneumonia may include progressive and severe respiratory distress or a bimodal, delayed deterioration. Physical or radiographic signs of pneumonia are of urgent importance. Historically, bacterial superinfections following influenza have prominently involved *Haemophilus influenzae* (so-named because it was found so commonly in the lungs of those stricken with the "Spanish" flu), *Staphylococcus aureus*, and *Streptococcus pneumoniae*. However, all varieties of bacteria may be involved and clinicians should be aggressive in identifying potential bacterial pathogens for targeted antibiotic coverage. The complication of bacterial pneumonia following influenza is particularly dangerous in older patients with co-morbidities such as chronic obstructive pulmonary disease (COPD) and congestive heart failure (CHF).

Treatment

For the treatment of patients with particularly severe or complicated influenza (pneumonia, myositis/myoglobinuria, and encephalopathy), antiviral agents may be employed. These agents (Table 3-2) have been shown to lessen the severity and duration of influenzal illness. They may also be used as prophylactic agents against influenza A (H_1N_1, H_2N_2, H_3N_2, and H_5N_1) strains. They might be used most reasonably among the elderly to prevent illness or limit the severity of disease. However, all of these drugs have side effects and should not be employed casually.

Amantadine (Symmetrel) and rimantadine (Flumadine) are related agents that have been used for a number of years, whereas oseltamivir (TamiFlu) and zanamivir (Relenza) are newer agents. Rimantadine has fewer side effects and is generally preferred over amantadine in the elderly. Zanamivir, an inhaled agent, has been greatly limited in its use due to airway

Table 3-2 Antiviral Agents for Influenza Treatment or Prevention in Adults

Agent	Route/Dose	Side Effects/Toxicity
Amantadine (Influenza A only) Trade name: Symmetrel	• Oral (tablet, capsule, syrup) • <65 yo = 100 mg bid • ≥65 yo = <100 mg bid	• More side effects than rimantadine • Reduce dose with impaired renal function • Anxiety, confusion, seizures
Rimantadine (Influenza A only) Trade name: Flumadine	• Oral (tablet, syrup) • <65 yo = 100 mg bid • ≥65 yo = 100 or 200 mg daily	• Fewer side effects than amantadine • Cleared via liver, not kidneys
Oseltamivir (Influenza A & B) Trade name: Tamiflu	• Oral (capsule, suspension) • 75 mg bid	• Nausea, vomiting
Zanamivir (Influenza A & B) Trade name: Relenza	• Inhalation only • 2 inhalations bid	• May cause severe bronchospasm; a problem for those with chronic asthma or acute airway reactivity to influenza

reactivity. Unlike the former agents, which are active only versus A strains, oseltamivir and zanamivir are useful against both A and B disease.

High resistance to amantadine and rimantadine in the new highly feared H_5N_1 bird flu viruses has been reported, so these agents cannot be relied upon for either prevention or modification of avian influenza. So far there have been only two reported cases that were resistant to oseltamivir (TamiFlu). Presently, there is debate about personal stockpiling of this valuable agent. These infections occurred in victims in early 2005 and have not been reported elsewhere. Fears of misuse and resulting widespread resistance have been voiced. The resistant strain was identified in July 2005, but as of late summer 2006 no further evidence of H_5N_1 resistance has been found (Brett and Zuger 2005). Zanamivir resistance has not been reported. It is unknown whether the resistant strain of H_5N_1 has virulence equal to the wild strain. However, human-to-human spread of H_5N_1 has not occurred as of the time of this writing.

Prevention

We may visualize prevention in terms of three broad strategies: *vaccination*, *antiviral therapy*, and *avoidance and hygiene*. In rare instances, anti-influenzal agents or chemotherapy may be given for prevention to high-risk persons who have not been vaccinated against (or for) influenza.

Vaccination

All persons 65 years of age and older should receive the influenza vaccine annually. The only respiratory tract viral infection for which there is a vaccine is influenza. However, vaccination has been problematic due to the antigenic variability related to the presence of two major strains, influenza A and B, and—more important—antigenic "drift" as well as "shift" within these strains (see section on "Influenza" for more details). Influenza C viruses are rarely associated with epidemic disease and are not included in vaccines. Currently, inactivated vaccines are generally employed (rather than living "attenuated" strains) in the United States. However, a new live vaccine is now licensed for persons aged 5 to 50, "FluMist" (MedImmune, Gaithersburg, Maryland). Given by nasal instillation, it has theoretical advantages but neither its efficacy nor safety has been demonstrated in the elderly. Persons for whom flu vaccines are to be given are listed in Table 3-3.

Antiviral therapy—amantadine and rimantadine—are not reliable against H_5N_1 flu strains. Oseltamivir (TamiFlu) and zanamivir (Relenza) have been effective thus far. Stockpiling of these agents for future use is controversial, but it is commonly done in the United States, particularly TamiFlu.

The primary humoral immunogenic determinants of the influenza viruses are the *hemagglutinin* (HA) and *neuraminidase* (NA) components of the cell walls. Viruses and vaccines are commonly designated by their HA and NA patterns. The major challenge for vaccine production in North America is to anticipate which virus(es) will be epidemic in a forthcoming winter. To do this, there is an ongoing surveillance program in the Orient where the new strains appear to evolve, due in large measure to proximity of large human

Table 3-3 Groups for Whom Influenza Vaccination is Indicated

A. Persons older than 50 years (this has been modified to 65 years or older during times of vaccine shortage)

B. Persons at increased risk for complications:

    1. Those with chronic respiratory or cardiovascular disorders including asthma

    2. Immunosuppressed persons including HIV-infection, organ transplantation, oncologic or rheumatologic chemotherapy, and chronic metabolic disorders including type 1 diabetes mellitus, renal failure, and hemoglobinopathies

C. Persons who can transmit influenza to those at high risk:

    1. Physicians, nurses, and other personnel in hospital or outpatient care facilities

    2. Employees of nursing homes or other chronic care facilities including assisted-living and home-care programs

    3. Families in contact with high-risk elderly

populations to swine and avian species wherein mutated and hybrid viruses devolve. Each year, authorities in the West attempt to estimate which viruses are most likely to be epidemic and how many doses of vaccine will be appropriate for the groups at risk.

The vaccines are to be given to susceptible subjects in North America in the fall of the year, typically between September and mid-November. Flu vaccines have been designated as "whole virus" (WV) or "split virus" (SV); in the United States SV products are primarily employed.

The Centers for Disease Control conducted a case-controlled study of vaccine effectiveness in Colorado in 2003-2004 that was highly instructive. That flu season was marked by the early appearance of disease, severe illness, and circulation of a strain of influenza A, H_3N_2, that was not well matched by the year's vaccine (although it was an H_3N_2 vaccine) (CDC 2004). It has been estimated that ordinarily the vaccine would confer a 70-90% protection in adults less than 65 years of age when it is well-matched against the dominant seasonal strain. Its efficacy in those older than 65 years of age is 50% to 60% in terms of preventing respiratory illness, pneumonia, and hospitalization. In 2003-2004, the vaccine yielded 38-52% protection against laboratory confirmed influenza in adults. Today there are massive efforts underway to produce an effective H_5N_1 vaccine agent for the feared "bird flu" that began in 2005 and is rapidly advancing amongst chickens and other birds.

Antiviral Therapy

When influenza is raging in a community and a clinician is confronted with a patient who failed to receive the vaccine previously, several steps may be taken. The vaccine should be given, even belatedly. It takes approximately 2 to 4 weeks for protective antibody levels to form. Meanwhile, if a particularly vulnerable individual is intimately exposed to flu, one can commence prophylactic therapy with one of the newer antivirals, oseltamivir or zanamivir (see Table 3-3).

Avoidance and Hygiene

For the elderly in general and for the fragile elderly in particular (underlying lung or cardiovascular disease or immunocompromised), it is prudent to limit social contacts during a community outbreak of influenza. While the common cold is most often spread by direct physical contact, influenza is usually spread by aerosols generated by coughing or sneezing. During the peak seasons, one should counsel the elderly to (*a*) limit social gatherings, (b) be cautious regarding hand-shaking and embracing, (c) avoid sharing glasses, utensils and food/drink, and (d) minimize contact with shared objects such as doorknobs or faucets. Frequent hand-washing (or use of cleansing lotions that do not require water) may be helpful, although no controlled studies have proven this. Perhaps the greatest challenge for the elderly may be to limit their exposure to, and contact with, grandchildren. Although "adorable," youngsters should be seen as viral-vectors *par excellence*.

Questions may arise about the efficacy of masks or so-called respirators. In general such devices are not regularly worn, do not fit well, cause discomfort (especially among those with underlying lung disease), and have not been proven efficacious.

Severe Acute Respiratory Syndrome

Severe acute respiratory syndrome (SARS) was a designation for a new, frequently lethal viral illness that arose in China and spread via human travel to other communities including a dramatic outbreak in Toronto, Canada. Due to its novelty and relatively high lethality (up to 15%), including health-care workers, it received great public attention in 2003-2004 (Lau et al 2004). However, it caused far less morbidity and mortality than did influenza and may or may not reappear in subsequent years. Prevention involves avoiding travel to endemic areas and avoidance of both direct physical contact and aerosol exposure. Health care workers with both intensive and prolonged contact to diseased individuals appeared to be at particular risk, and universal precautions as well as ventilation measures appear appropriate.

The SARS virus represents a novel mutation of the corona-virus family, traditional agents of "the common cold." It may have evolved through animal vectors which have intimate contacts with Asian populations. Efforts are underway to develop a vaccine.

Summary

Viral illnesses involving both the upper and lower respiratory tracts are common among the elderly, producing significant morbidity and—in the cases of influenza and SARS—posing lethal threats. Influenza vaccination is an essential element of health maintenance for adults. Antiviral drugs may be used to attenuate the severity or, in some cases, to prevent the flu. Avoidance strategies may be helpful in lessening the risk of viral infections of the respiratory tract.

BIBLIOGRAPHY AND SUGGESTED READING

Barry JM. The Great Influenza. New York: Viking; 2004. *A full-length volume describing the background behind the 1918 influenza pandemic and the nature of influenza epidemics. This story is intertwined with the personalities that drove modern medical science in the 20th century.*

Brett AS, Zuger A. The run on Tamiflu: should physicians prescribe on demand? N Engl J Med. 2005;353:2636-7. *This is an editorial expressing concern over the widespread prescribing and stockpiling of oseltamivir. This issue contains the first report of two cases of oseltamivir resistance and a commentary on the mechanisms of resistance.*

Centers for Disease Control and Prevention. Assessment of the effectiveness of the 2003-04 influenza vaccine among children and adults—Colorado, 2003. MMWR Morbidity and Mortality Weekly Report 2004;53:707-10 (August 13). *This case-controlled study documents the effectiveness of the 2003-4 vaccine in both the elderly and young populations in Colorado. It was a valuable lesson in a state in which there are relatively high rates of vaccination, demonstrating modest protection despite a suboptimal match versus the dominant influenza strain that year.*

Lau JTF, Yang X, Leung P-C, et al. SARS in three categories of hospital workers, Hong Kong. Emerg Infect Dis. 2004;10:1399-1404. *The authors characterize the risk factors for nosocomial transmission to health care workers, noting the particular risk for clerical and cleaning staffs on the wards.*

Sethi S. Bacterial pneumonia: managing a deadly complication of influenza in older adults with comorbid disease. Geriatrics. 2002;57:56-61.

Svoboda T, Henry B, Shulman L, et al. Public health measures to control the spread of the severe acute respiratory syndrome during the outbreak in Toronto. N Engl J Med. 2004;350:2352-61. *Documents the nature of the SARS outbreak and the efficacy of measures taken including quarantine. Although focused upon SARS, such measures may well be appropriate/needed were there to be an epidemic of a highly lethal ("shifted") variety of influenza.*

Weinstein RA. Planning for epidemics—the lessons of SARS. N Engl J Med. 2004;350:2332-35. *Examines the various settings in which the SARS epidemic was confronted and discusses the preventive measures employed.*

Yu ITS, Yuguo L, Wong TW, et al. Evidence of airborne transmission of the severe acute respiratory syndrome virus. N Engl J Med. 2004;350:1731-39. *Documents airborne spread of SARS in Hong Kong, helping to clarify the "mysterious" epidemiological pattern of the original outbreak.*

4 Community-Acquired Pneumonia

ommunity-acquired pneumonia (CAP) in adults, including the geriatric population, remains a common but serious respiratory disease. It occurs more commonly in the winter months but can occur at any time, and has a significant morbidity, mortality, and economic impact on the population. The cost of CAP in the United States has been estimated at $20 billion annually. Among the geriatric population, there are many similarities to younger-adult CAP cases, although specific circumstances, such as aspiration risk, nursing home residence, comorbid diseases, and social factors may be associated with specific pathogens and may influence decisions regarding treatment regimens, duration of treatment, and whether hospitalization is necessary.

Although there have been numerous articles, opinions, investigational studies, and consensus guidelines published in the past 10 years, there has even been debate on basics such as testing, therapy, and criteria for hospitalization.

This chapter summarizes the diagnosis and treatment of CAP in the elderly, and treatment of non-ICU hospitalized patients. Treatment of nursing home acquired pneumonia is covered in Chapter 6.

Pathogens

The organism responsible for CAP is identified specifically in only about 50% of patients, even under the most intense hospital-based efforts of physicians. The office-based physician has much less practical testing available. Nonetheless, the most common pathogens in outpatients with CAP are *Streptococcus pneumoniae, Chlamydia pneumoniae, Legionella* spp., and

Haemophilus influenzae. Other, less common organisms, including viruses, can also be etiologic factors. In fact, these pathogens are the same as those most commonly involved in ICU and non-ICU hospitalized patients. However, other pathogens can exist in hospitalized patients (Blasi 2004). Because cultures for specific organisms are not usually obtained in outpatients, we only need to be aware of the most common pathogens for treatment options and guidelines.

Some exceptions to consider include *Klebsiella pneumoniae* with alcoholics, anaerobic organisms in elderly potential aspirators, and increased incidence of *Haemophilus influenzae* and *Moraxella catarrhalis* in smokers and COPD patients. Age alone, in the absence of comorbid illness, has little impact on the bacterial etiology of CAP.

Atypical pathogens include *Chlamydia pneumoniae*, *Mycoplasma pneumoniae*, and *Legionella* spp. Current thought is that atypical pneumonia presents with the same signs and symptoms as other bacterial agents causing CAP.

Pneumococcal Resistance

Much has been written about penicillin-resistant *Streptococcus pneumoniae,* an increasing problem, especially in localized areas of the country, which must not be ignored. The antibiotics whose administration has been associated with acquired resistance to the pneumococcus are primarily penicillin, trimethoprim-sulfamethoxazole (Bactrim), tetracycline, and, to some degree, macrolides.

The clinical relevance of drug-resistant pneumococcus has been debated, and most investigators have found no difference in mortality for patients infected with resistant or sensitive organisms, after controlling for comorbid illness. Nonetheless, this may become a more significant problem in the future. A few factors that increase the risk of infections with drug-resistant pneumococci are:

- Age greater than 65
- Beta-lactam therapy within the past 3 months
- Alcoholism
- Immune-suppressive illness (including corticosteroid therapy)
- Multiple medical comorbidities
- Exposure to a child in a daycare center
- Recent hospitalization

Diagnosis

A useful algorithm for the patient presenting to the office for cough suggestive of CAP is shown in Figure 4-1. Elderly patients may not present with many of the usual signs and symptoms such as fever, cough, and sputum production;

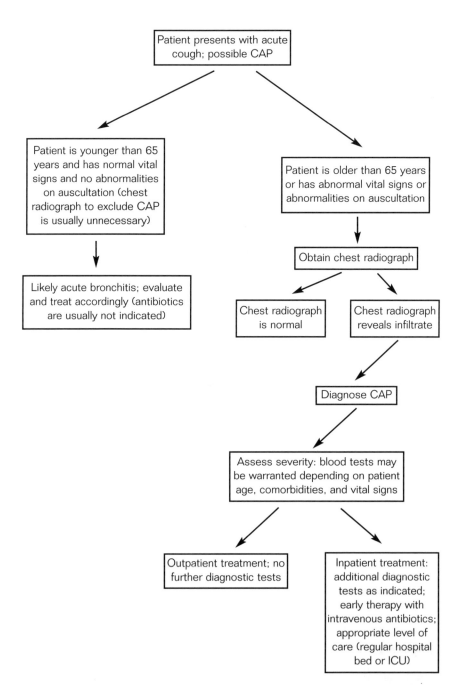

Figure 4-1 Diagnostic evaluation of community-acquired pneumonia. (Adapted from Frazee BW. Community-acquired pneumonia: getting down to the basics. J Respir Dis. 2004;25.)

therefore, a low threshold for hospitalization is advised for these patients. The diagnosis of CAP should always include a chest radiograph. Any diagnosis without a radiograph is more of an educated guess and may lead to undue problems. Sputum cultures are impractical in the office and are not recommended by the American Thoracic Society. Blood cultures and CBC are likewise impractical, expensive, and probably will not affect the treatment of the office patient.

Emergency room evaluation may include CBC, blood cultures, assessment of oxygenation, and usually sputum culture, although, again, the value of a sputum culture has been questioned. Gram stain of sputum may occasionally be useful to broaden antibiotic coverage for organisms found on the Gram stain that are not covered by usual initial antibiotic therapy.

Determining whether a patient with CAP should be hospitalized is one of the most critical decisions facing the office-based physician. There are at least five guidelines on risk factors or comorbidity with value scales to aid hospitalization and treatment decisions. Unfortunately, such guidelines are sometimes overly complex. Furthermore, analysis of the patient with CAP cannot depend solely on a list of comorbidities but must also involve the "art of medicine," evaluating not only comorbidities but also the amount of involvement as shown by x-ray, presence of pleural effusion, general strength of the patient, quality of the home, and social considerations such as available help for meal preparation. The decision on whether to hospitalize also includes factors such as medications, nausea, dehydration, weakness, fever, respiratory rate, blood pressure, hypoxemia, confusion, and extrapulmonary sites of possible infection.

Hospitalization should be considered in patients with any of the following risk factors:

- Age 65 or older
- COPD
- Diabetes mellitus
- Renal insufficiency
- Congestive heart failure
- Coronary heart disease
- Chronic neurological conditions
- Chronic liver disease

Treatment

Selecting the appropriate treatment may be the most confusing aspect of CAP. Expert opinion in the United States, Europe, and Canada differs slightly. Most clinicians rely primarily on the American Thoracic Society (ATS) guidelines, but other guidelines are also used. Treatment varies depending on clinical setting (outpatient, hospital, ICU), presence of comorbidities, route of antibiotic administration (oral or IV), and length of therapy. This chapter does not discuss ICU treatment, which is more complicated. Empiric treatment choices based on clinical setting and presence of comorbidities are shown in Table 4-1.

Duration of treatment is debatable, but the consensus is 7-10 days. Infection with an atypical pathogen, if suspected, should be treated for 10-14 days. Patients on corticosteroids may require 14 days or longer.

Whether to treat orally or intravenously is also debatable. Oral outpatient treatment is obviously easier, although intravenous antibiotics can usually be arranged. Oral treatment with doxycycline, macrolides, amoxicillin-clavulanate, or respiratory quinolones seems to cover a good spectrum of pathogens with little or no resistance. (However, although one may be tempted to conclude that oral respiratory quinolones will cover all organisms of concern, it is best not to overuse an antibiotic; over-treatment and drug resistance may result.) Inpatient treatment is usually intravenous antibiotics. However, there is good evidence that oral antipneumococcal fluoroquinolones may be given even for hospitalized patients, provided their gastrointestinal tracts are functional. Azithromycin is as effective orally and intravenously. A switch to oral administration in 24-48 hours is appropriate if the patient is clinically improving and the gastrointestinal tract is functional. The patient may be discharged on the same day that oral antibiotics are started.

Table 4-1 Antibiotic Choices for Community-Acquired Pneumonia

Outpatient Treatment

No major comorbidity	Macrolide (azithromycin [Zithromax] or clarithromycin [Biaxin]) or doxycycline
Comorbidity	B-lactam (cefuroxime [Ceftin]), high-dose amoxicillin, Augmentin (amoxicillin/clavulanate) and macrolide or doxycycline
	or
	Antipneumococcal fluoroquinolone alone (levofloxacin [Levaquin]), gatifloxacin [Tequin], moxifloxacin [Avelox])

Hospital Treatment (Non-ICU)

No major comorbidity	Azithromycin (IV or PO) or doxycycline plus B-lactam
	or
	Antipneumococcal fluoroquinolone
Comorbidity	Same as Comorbidity Outpatient Treatment above (but larger choice of B-lactams if patient on IV)

Recent studies have shown that high-dose short-course levofloxacin (Levaquin) (750 mg daily for 5 days) and the standard dose (500 mg daily for 10 days) are equally effective for mild-to-severe CAP (Dunbar et al 2003).

If there is a high suspicion of pneumococcal resistance, the Centers for Disease Control (CDC) has suggested oral cefuroxime (Ceftin), amoxicillin-clavulanate 875 mg bid, IV ceftriaxone, or an antipneumococcal fluoroquinolone. Several other antibiotics are also effective. Vancomycin and linezolid (Zyvox) should be reserved for patients with high-level resistance.

If no improvement in the patient's condition is seen after 3 to 4 days of treatment, the clinician should reconsider the diagnosis or consider hospitalizing the patient, as appropriate.

Prevention

Pneumococcal vaccination works and is cost effective (Christenson et al 2004). Current recommendations are that all patients over 65 years of age should receive vaccinations, and patients under 65 should be vaccinated if they have a chronic disease. A single revaccination is indicated in patients over age 65 if they received the vaccine more than 5 years earlier and were younger than 65 when they got their first dose. If patients were older than age 65 when they got their first dose, one is enough.

Summary

The following checklist may be used for CAP evaluation in the geriatric office patient:

- Evaluate the patient thoroughly.
- Obtain a chest radiograph.
- Consider comorbidities.
- Consider potential for pneumococcal resistance.
- Decide whether the patient needs hospitalization.
- Choose an appropriate therapeutic regimen.
- Reconsider diagnosis and/or hospitalize the patient if no improvement in 3-4 days.

The treatment programs discussed previously are appropriate at present. We must, however, be aware that as new antibiotics appear and resistant organisms develop, treatment recommendations will change.

BIBLIOGRAPHY AND SUGGESTED READING

American Thoracic Society. Guidelines for the Management of Adults with Community-Acquired Pneumonia: Diagnoses, Assessment of Severity, Antimicrobial Therapy, and Prevention. Am J Respir Crit Care Med. 2001;163:1730-54. *Probably the gold standard for CAP management. Provides excellent information on all aspects of CAP.*

Blasi F. Atypical pathogens and respiratory tract infections. Eur Respir J. 2004;24:171-81. *Discusses European guidelines for the management of CAP and the importance of atypical pathogens.*

Christenson B, Hedlund J, Lundberg P, et al. Additive preventive effect of influenza and pneumococcal vaccines in elderly persons. Eur Respir J. 2004;23:363-8. *The use of both vaccines was effective in preventing the need for hospitalization for both influenza and pneumonia and decreasing the overall incidence of both.*

Cunha BA. Empiric therapy of community-acquired pneumonia: guidelines for the perplexed. Chest. 2004;125:1913-9. *Somewhat controversial regarding therapeutic options, although a good review. Suggests avoiding macrolides because of S. pneumoniae resistance.*

Dunbar LM, Wunderink RG, Habib MP, et al. High-dose, short-course levofloxacin for community-acquired pneumonia: a new treatment paradigm. Clin Infect Dis. 2003:37;752-60. *A new approach with high-dose levofloxacin therapy.*

File TM, Garau J, Blasi F, et al. Guidelines for empiric antimicrobial prescribing in community-acquired pneumonia. Chest. 2004;125:1888-1901. *Pertinent update on treatment with discussion about differences in American and European guidelines. Discusses the differences between various guidelines by societies other than the American Thoracic Society.*

Frazee BW. Community-acquired pneumonia: getting down to the basics. J Respir Dis. 2004;25.

Houck PM, Bratzler DW, Nsa W, et al. Timing of antibiotic administration and outcomes for Medicare patients hospitalized with community-acquired pneumonia. Arch Intern Med. 2004;164:637-44. *Early use of antibiotics is associated with a favorable outcome.*

Mylotte JM, Ksiazek S, Bentley DW. Rational approach to the antibiotic treatment of pneumonia in the elderly. Drugs Aging. 1994;4:21-33. *Useful state-of-the-art review.*

5 Hospital-Acquired Pneumonia

ospital-acquired pneumonia (HAP), or nosocomial pneumonia, is a serious complication of hospitalized patients. HAP is associated with increased mortality, increased morbidity including prolongation of hospital stay, and increased economic costs. Many of the same risk factors that predispose elderly people to community-acquired pneumonia (CAP) also put them at risk for HAP. Nevertheless, it is not clear whether increasing age itself is an important independent risk factor for HAP. Studies have found mixed results on this question. In fact, one of the largest cohort studies, using a computerized system database available in several hospitals for studying ventilator-associated pneumonia (VAP), a major component of HAP, found that patients developing VAP were statistically significantly younger than those who did not develop HAP, although the actual difference in mean age, 61.7 versus 64.6 years respectively, was not very great (Rello et al 2002). This result is somewhat surprising because the other risk factors associated with HAP in most studies are conditions that might be expected to increase with age and are similar to the risk conditions for CAP.

Although there are several studies focusing on CAP in the elderly, this is not the case for HAP. Until better information is available, therefore, the approach to and the management of HAP in the elderly are the same as for HAP in other patients, with a few exceptions that will be described.

Definitions

Some people have divided HAP into early (usually occurring within 5 days of admission to hospital) and late (occurring after 5 days). Opinions differ as to whether the organisms involved in early versus late pneumonia are different. Authors who emphasize a difference in the pathogenic flora argue that HAP should be defined as occurring after some arbitrary time from admission to hospital, often after 5-7 days. These authors claim that any pneumonia occurring before that time is likely secondary to community-acquired organisms colonizing the patient before hospital admission. Therefore, they argue that patients with pneumonia developing during the first several days of hospitalization should be considered as having CAP and managed according to the guidelines for that condition.

Epidemiology

HAP is the second most common nosocomial infection in hospitalized patients, after urinary tract infections. The incidence has been reported to be about 1% of all hospitalizations but varies considerably with the demographics and co-morbidities of the patient population studied. In a large 1-day point prevalence study of 10,000 mechanically ventilated patients in European ICUs, 10% of patients had HAP at that point in time (Rello et al 2002). Another large study, in 107 European ICUs, found a similar prevalence of 9% for VAP, with a three-fold higher risk of developing HAP in ventilated than in non-ventilated critically ill patients. Other studies have shown a 3- to 21-fold higher rate of pneumonia for ventilated compared with non-ventilated critically ill patients (Rello et al 2001). The above figures of 10% and 9% represent a point prevalence; that is, at a single given point in time, about 10% of ICU patients had HAP. When the VAP incidence (VAP development at any time during the hospitalization) is studied, the figures are higher with an incidence of usually 20-28%. VAP incidence is higher in patients with acute lung injury (ALI) and/or acute respiratory distress syndrome (ARDS) than in other ventilated patients. Whereas the mortality for nosocomial infections involving the urinary tract or skin is relatively low, ranging from 1-4%, the mortality rate for VAP is substantial, ranging from 24-50%, or in some studies even higher. The prognosis tends to be worse for patients with gram-negative bacilli as the pathogenic organism than for those with gram-positive bacteria.

Morbidity and excess costs are also associated with nosocomial pneumonia. This has been best studied in VAP. Several studies suggest that duration of mechanical ventilation, ICU length of stay, and hospital length of stay are 25-100% longer in patients with VAP than in matched control subjects without VAP.

Several risk factors have been associated with HAP. Again, this has been much better studied in VAP than in HAP in general. These risk factors can roughly be divided into two groups: host factors and factors associated with medical interventions. Regarding host factors, as mentioned above, some studies have found increasing age, particularly greater than age 60, to be an independent risk factor, but others have not. Poor nutritional status reflected by a serum albumin of less than 2.2 is associated with a higher incidence of VAP. Several underlying risk conditions, including ALI and ARDS, COPD, coma, burns, trauma, and multi-organ failure, are associated with higher risks of pneumonia. Chronic comorbid conditions carry a higher risk, and the influence of comorbidity and the underlying risk condition may explain why age may not be found to be an independent variable in some of the studies. Studies using scales that attempt to assess severity of illness find that higher severity of illness is associated with a higher incidence of VAP. Large-volume gastric aspiration is clearly associated with increased incidence of HAP, but it is likely that small amounts of aspiration are also associated because it has been shown that gastric, upper respiratory, or tracheal colonization is a risk for nosocomial pneumonia.

Management factors associated with increased risk for pneumonia may be related to the therapy itself, to the interventions, or may simply reflect greater severity of illness or some of the already mentioned underlying risk conditions. Mechanical ventilation for longer than 2 days is one of the intervention factors. Reintubation is associated with an increased risk of VAP. Antacids as a treatment for preventing stress ulceration are associated with increased risk of pneumonia, but the status of other prophylactic stress ulcer therapy is less clear. Most studies suggest that H2 blockers carry a higher risk of pneumonia than sucralfate. However, one of the largest and best-conducted studies failed to find this difference. The supine position is strongly associated with increased risk for pneumonia, probably because of the propensity for aspiration (Drakulovic et al 1999). (This will be discussed further in the Prevention section.) Other interventions associated with increased risk of pneumonia include the use of paralytic agents, continuous as opposed to bolus or interrupted intravenous sedation, administration of more than 4 units of blood products, the presence of a nasogastric tube, and previous antibiotic therapy.

Pathogenesis

Some aspects of HAP pathogenesis remain speculative, but most investigators believe that the major pathogenetic mechanism is the micro-aspiration of colonized upper airway or gastric secretions. It has been known since the early 1970s that with the onset of critical illness, there is a change over several days in the flora of the stomach and the upper airway, with potential pathogens appearing in the stomach, the mouth, and perhaps even the trachea. This is in part related to changes in the quality of the cells in the upper airway which make the surface of the cell stickier, predisposing to pathogens adhering to the mucosal cell surface. HAP can also occur by the bloodborne route related to intravenous line infections or other causes of bacteremia.

Modern endotracheal tubes use a high-volume and low-pressure cuff or balloon, which helps to prevent mucosal injury to the trachea at the site of the tube cuff. However, this allows small quantities of secretions to continuously leak through small invaginations of the cuff, where it does not fit perfectly in the airway. Thus, it is likely that small amounts of secretions above the cuff leak into the lower airway and contaminate the lower airway with the altered flora present in the upper airway. Changes in gastric colonization often precede the changes in upper airway colonization. Therefore, much of the effort to prevent HAP has been focused on preventing the colonization of the stomach, and thus of the upper airway, as well as preventing larger amounts of aspiration from occurring, primarily by keeping the patient in a semi-recumbent position.

Diagnosis

As in CAP, HAP in elderly patients may present in unusual ways, especially with a change in mental status, and may not have other typical findings, such as fever, that readily indicate pneumonia. Therefore a high degree of suspicion for HAP in the elderly must be maintained.

Diagnosis of HAP can be difficult. Although, obviously, a new infiltrate on chest X-ray, fever, purulent sputum production, and increased white blood cell count should suggest the development of HAP, unfortunately most of these findings are not specific and occur in many other conditions. This is particularly true of fever and leukocytosis. Sputum production, although somewhat more specific, certainly is not limited to pneumonia. Furthermore, the more critically ill the patient, the more difficult the diagnosis. Many hospitalized patients may already have pulmonary infiltrates on chest x-rays, making the appreciation of new infiltrates difficult.

Making a diagnosis of VAP is especially problematic in patients with ALI or ARDS. These patients have preexisting diffuse infiltrates, making it very difficult to appreciate changes in a chest x-ray that may represent a new pneumonia. At the same time, it is well established that the inflammatory condition of ALI/ARDS can cause fever, leukocytosis, and purulent pulmonary secretions. These issues make the study of HAP and VAP difficult because there is no gold standard for diagnosis. The situation has been made clearer in VAP through multiple studies evaluating the use of quantitative cultures obtained by BAL and PSB through a fiberoptic bronchoscope. These have led to the conclusion that quantitative cultures can be useful in identifying patients with pneumonia.

Treatment

Although *Streptococcus pneumoniae* is one of the causative organisms of HAP, it is a less common etiology in HAP than in CAP. *Staphylococcus aureus,* including methicillin-resistant *S. aureus* (MRSA), and gram-negative bacilli, including *Pseudomonas* and *Acinetobacter*, which tend to be resistant to some antibiotics, are greatly increased in the etiology of HAP compared with CAP. However, much more important than this general information is knowledge about the incidence and antibiotic resistance pattern of microorganisms causing HAP in each institution. Considerable variability exists among hospitals and geographic regions in both the likely organisms for HAP and their antibiotic resistance. Therefore, although general guidelines can be used as a starting point, it is necessary to adapt these guidelines to the patterns found in a particular institution.

The general treatment guidelines essentially are based on whether or not resistant *Pseudomonas* and *Acinetobacter* or MRSA is likely to be causing the HAP in the individual institution and patient (American Thoracic Society 2005). If these organisms are not likely to be responsible, one can treat the other likely organisms with any of several options (American Thoracic Society 2005): ceftiraxone; a quinolone such as levofloxacin, moxifloxacin, or ciptorfloxacin; ampicillin-sulbactam; or ertapenem. On the other hand, in the more likely case of multi-drug resistant organisms such as *Pseudomonas* or *Acinetobacter* (which are of particular concern), double coverage is recommended with a beta-lactam plus either an antipseudomonal fluoroguinolone (ciprofloxacin or levoflaxacin) or an aminoglycoside. Suggested options for the beta-lactam include: an antipseudomonal cephalosporin such as cefepime or ceftazidime; an antipseudomonal carbapenem such as imipenem or meropenem; or a beta-lactam/beta-lactamase inhibitor such as piperacillin-tazobactam.

If MRSA is a consideration, vancomycin can be added. One of the above antibiotic choices should be started as empiric therapy, but if quantitative cultures have been obtained, the treatment can be tailored to the predominant organism grown once the cultures are available. Again, if the quantitative cultures are negative (i.e., if they fall below the accepted cutoffs for the diagnosis of pneumonia), antibiotics can be discontinued, although this obviously requires some clinical judgment. If pneumonia is considered unlikely by a low quantitative culture growth, infections in other sites should be considered and appropriate diagnostic studies performed.

Prevention

Several strategies have been suggested to reduce the incidence of HAP. These strategies have usually been tested regarding VAP, but the data may be extrapolated in some cases to patients at risk for HAP but not receiving mechanical ventilation. Most of these strategies have been tested in relatively small trials and do not reach the level of IA evidence, the highest level of evidence basis. However, some of the strategies have been found to have consistent positive results in smaller studies and, because they are not associated with toxicity and are inexpensive, they can be recommended for implementation.

The most important strategy for reducing VAP appears to be keeping the patient in the semi-recumbent rather than recumbent position. Three trials have evaluated the efficacy of this approach. It has been previously shown that supine positioning is independently associated with the development of VAP, presumably because of increased risk of esophageal reflux and aspiration. The trials have tested elevating the head of the bed to 45 degrees. Two trials measured gastroesophageal reflux and aspiration events as surrogate outcomes and showed a decreased frequency in both of these outcomes. The third trial found a statistically significant reduction in VAP in patients nursed with the head of the bed elevated to 45 degrees compared with those maintained in the supine position. There was no difference in mortality in this relatively small study. Because there were no adverse effects observed in patients randomly assigned to the semi-recumbent position and because this is a low-cost, low-risk strategy, it is recommended that all patients in the critical care unit be kept in a semi-recumbent position unless there is a specific contraindication. Contraindications might include particular types of recent surgery or shock refractory to vasoactive therapy. Although this is a simple strategy, it can be difficult to implement in all patients in whom it is indicated. It requires cooperation, especially by the nurses who need to understand both the rationale for the strategy and its potential importance. This involves education of the physicians, nurses, and respiratory therapists, but also requires leadership by all three of these groups.

Patients who are mechanically ventilated are known to be at risk for stress gastric ulceration. Data from the 1980s suggested that antacids and possibly H2 blockers, which reduce the gastric acidity in an attempt to decrease stress ulceration, were associated with increased risk for VAP. Sucralfate, which protects the mucosa from stress ulceration but does not affect the gastric pH, was found to have lower rates of VAP. Several other studies also found that sucralfate was superior to H2 blockers in reducing the incidence of VAP. However, a more recent large well-designed trial of 1200 mechanically ventilated patients found that H2 blockers were more effective than sucralfate in preventing clinically important gastrointestinal bleeding and failed to find a significant difference in the VAP between these two (Collard et al, Ann Intern Med, 2003). H2 blockers are more expensive than sucralfate, but they are easier to administer. Therefore, with our current state of knowledge, one can choose between H2 blockers or sucralfate to prevent stress ulceration in mechanically ventilated patients.

Continuous or intermittent aspiration of (i.e., removal of) pooled secretions above the endotracheal tube cuff has been suggested to reduce VAP development. This requires the use of specially designed endotracheal tubes with a suction port above the cuff. This method has been studied in small trials with results that are mixed but generally favorable. However, because of the mixed results and the small numbers of studies, this approach needs to be studied further before it can be recommended for routine use.

Several studies of beds that rotate the position of the patient (so-called oscillating beds) have been performed. A meta-analysis of six of these randomized controlled trials found a statistically significant reduction in the risk for pneumonia, but five of these studies were limited to surgical patients or patients with neurologic impairment. The sixth study, which was primarily in medical ICU patients, found no significant benefit. The cost of these beds is relatively expensive. However, there is reasonable evidence that this practice may be effective in selected surgical patients or patients with neurological problems. Further studies in medical ICU patients should be done before use of oscillating beds can be recommended.

Several studies have looked at the frequency of changing ventilator circuits. In general, more frequent changes are associated with a higher incidence of colonization, although there was no difference in the rate of VAP. Based on these findings, ventilator circuits can be changed less frequently based on the monitoring of colonization, with cost savings in addition to the lower incidence of colonization.

No clear evidence favors any specific form of enteral feeding in reducing VAP incidence.

BIBLIOGRAPHY AND SUGGESTED READING

American Thoracic Society and Infectious Diseases Society of America. Guidelines for the management of adults with hospital-acquired, ventilator-associated, and healthcare-associated pneumonia. Am J Respir Crit Care Med. 2005;171:388-416.

Chastre J, Fagon JY. Ventilator-associated pneumonia: state of the art. Am J Respir Crit Care Med. 2002;165:867-903. *Comprehensive review thoroughly discussing the issues involved in VAP.*

Chastre J, Wolff M, Fagon JY, et al. Comparison of 8 vs. 15 days of antibiotic therapy for ventilator-associated pneumonia in adults: a randomized trial. JAMA. 2003;290:2588-98. *Patients treated for 8 days compared with those treated for 15 days had neither excess mortality nor more recurrent infections, but they did have more mean antibiotic-free days. The authors concluded that with the possible exception of those with Pseudomonas pneumonias, there was comparable clinical effectiveness against VAP with the 8- and 15-day regimens and the 8-day group had less antibiotic use.*

Collard HR, Saint S, Matthay M. Prevention of ventilator-associated pneumonia: an evidence-based systematic review. Ann Intern Med. 2003;138:494-501. *Critical review of the literature for several strategies designed to reduce VAP.*

Cunha BA. Nosocomial pneumonia: diagnostic and therapeutic considerations. Med Clin North Am. 2001;85:79-114. *Review of diagnosis and management of nosocomial pneumonia in general (as opposed to VAP).*

Drakulovic MB, Torres A, Bauer TT, et al. Supine body position as a risk factor for nosocomial pneumonia in mechanically ventilated patients: a randomised trial. Lancet. 1999;354:1851-8. *This trial represents the best evidence for nursing all critically ill patients except for those with specific contraindications in a semi-recumbent position.*

Fagon JY, Chastre J, Wolff M, et al. Invasive and non-invasive strategies for management of suspected ventilator-associated pneumonia: a randomized trial. Ann Intern Med. 2000;132:621-30. *Patients receiving invasive management compared with patients managed clinically had a lower mortality, lower mean sepsis-related organ failure scores, and less antibiotic use.*

Ferrara AM, Fietta AM. New developments in antibacterial choice for lower respiratory tract infections in elderly patients. Drugs Aging. 2004;21:167-86. *Covers the recommendations for empiric therapy for HAP, but in particular discusses the influence of pharmacokinetics and drug interactions in the elderly upon these choices.*

Rello J, Ollendorf DA, Oster G, et al, for the VAP Outcomes Scientific Advisory Group. Epidemiology and outcomes of ventilator-associated pneumonia in a large US database. Chest. 2002;122:2115-21. *Demonstrates that VAP is a common nosocomial infection that is associated with poor clinical and economic outcomes. Notes that, while strategies to prevent the occurrence of VAP may not reduce mortality, they may yield other important benefits to patients, their families, and hospital systems.*

Rello J, Paiva JA, Baraibar J, et al. International Conference for the Development of Consensus on the Diagnosis and Treatment of Ventilator-Associated Pneumonia. Chest. 2001;120:955-70. *Consensus conference report attended by 12 investigators from Europe and Latin America to discuss strategies for the diagnosis and treatment of VAP.*

Tablan OC, Anderson LJ, Besser R, et al. Guidelines for preventing health-care-associated pneumonia, 2003. Recommendations of CDC and the Healthcare Infection Control Practices Advisory Committee. MMWR. 2004;53:1-36. *New guidelines designed to reduce the incidence of pneumonia in acute care hospitals. Available online at www.cdc.gov/mmwr/preview/mmwrhtml/rr5303a1.htm.*

6 Nursing Home Acquired Pneumonia

Pneumonia is the leading infectious cause of death in the United States and the fourth leading cause of mortality in persons over age 60. It has been estimated that up to 20% of patients hospitalized with pneumonia reside in either a nursing home or an extended care facility. Nursing home acquired pneumonia (NHAP) differs in many respects from CAP and HAP and should be considered a distinct entity.

Epidemiology

The incidence of pneumonia increases with age. The annual incidence is 91.6 per 100,000 for individuals under age 45; 277.2 per 100,000 for those aged 45 to 65; and 1012.3 per 100,000 for persons over age 65. A nursing home resident has a tenfold greater risk for developing pneumonia than a 75-year-old person living in the community. In anticipation of the continued growth of the nursing home population as our nation ages, it is estimated that 1.9 million nursing home residents will develop pneumonia annually over the next 30 years. Currently, one third of nursing home residents who are diagnosed with pneumonia will require hospital admission. The mortality for this group ranges from 20% to 40%.

Etiology

Infection from any cause is a common reason for deterioration of a nursing home resident's condition. A significant percentage of these patients require transfer to an acute care setting. Roughly 50% of these infections will involve the lung. Table 6-1 lists conditions often associated with increased risk of pneumonia among nursing home residents.

The decline in lung function that occurs with aging is one important predisposing factor for pneumonia. In addition, skeletal stiffening and calcification may be associated with a decreased effectiveness of cough. The decrease in the forced expiratory volume in 1 second that occurs with aging has been proven to be another important risk factor for severe pneumonia.

Immunosenescence, a well-known process on both an observational and a demonstrable laboratory basis, also contributes to the predisposition for infection in older persons. With the aging process, the ability to combat infection declines (see Chapter 1).

Aspiration probably represents the single most important risk factor for pneumonia in the elderly. The incidence of aspiration pneumonia in this group is reportedly three times that for age- and sex-matched individuals from the community. The incidence of aspiration increases when the patient's gag

Table 6-1 Risk Factors for Pneumonia in Nursing Home Residents

1. Decreased lung function

2. Bed-ridden status

3. Urinary incontinence

4. Age greater than 65

5. Male gender

6. Difficulty swallowing with increased risk of aspiration

   • Malnutrition

   • Tube feedings

   • Contractures

   • Hyperextended neck

   • Sedation/hypnotics

   • Anticholinergic medications

7. Underlying comorbid illness

   • COPD

   • Diabetes mellitus

   • Congestive heart failure

   • Neurologic disorders

   • Carcinoma

8. Enhanced oropharyngeal colonization (in response to recurrent antibiotic use)

reflex is impaired, mentation/consciousness levels are depressed, gastroe-sophageal reflux exists, or endotracheal tubes are in place. The aspiration may range from observed gastric acid aspiration to micro-aspiration of oropharyn-geal secretions, which most commonly is silent. Oropharyngeal colonization with aerobic gram-negative bacilli is seen in residents of nursing facilities, often exacerbated by repeated antibiotic usage that alters the normal flora. The common practice of using broad-spectrum antibiotics then aids the emer-gence of antibiotic resistance.

Finally, factors such as underlying comorbid illness (neurologic disorders, cardiac and pulmonary disease, diabetes) and common medications (seda-tives, psychoactive drugs) play an important role in the development of pneu-monia. Tuberculosis is often overlooked as a cause of NHAP. Whereas rates of tuberculosis in the elderly are twice that of the general population, they are four times higher among nursing home residents and 10-12 times that of the general population.

Identifying an etiologic pathogen in NHAP can be difficult. Few studies of NHAP have included extensive testing. The nursing home population often has poor cough effort and inability to cooperate with efforts to obtain sputum. When combined with the added problem of oropharyngeal colonization seen in the nursing home setting, establishing an etiologic agent becomes even more difficult. although the published percentages of etiologic agents differ from study to study, *Streptococcus pneumoniae* remains the most commonly identified organism. Table 6-2 lists pathogens commonly identified in NHAP.

Clinical Presentation

Classically it has been taught that the presentation of pneumonia in the nurs-ing home patient may be atypical and incompletely expressed. To a signifi-cant degree this can be attributed to coexisting illnesses. Compared with younger patients, nursing home residents have fewer classic symptoms of pneumonia such as cough, which is productive of purulent sputum, chills, and pleuritic chest pain. However, when compared with age-matched inde-pendent elderly, 75% of NHAP patients had fever and only 71% of CAP patients had fever. Cough was found less frequently in NHAP (63% vs. 81%), and dyspnea was also less common (39% vs. 46%). As would be expected in the elderly nursing home–confined patient, 75% were confused compared with only 37% of the elderly with CAP. In several studies of the manifesta-tions of NHAP, cough was present in 60% of the cases, dyspnea in 40%, fever in 65%, and an altered mental status in 50-70%. Additionally, an increased respiratory rate has been identified as a sensitive indicator of pneumonia and should be recognized.

Table 6-2 Pneumonia-Causing Pathogens Encountered in Nursing Homes

1. *Streptococcus pneumoniae*
   - Aspiration (aerobes and anaerobes)
2. Anerobic gram-negative bacilli
   - *Klebsiella*
   - *E. coli*
   - Others
3. *Staphylococcus aureus*
4. *Haemophilus influenzae*
5. *Moraxella catarrhalis*
6. *Mycobacterium tuberculosis*
7. *Chlamydia*
8. *Legionella*
9. *Mycoplasma*

Attention must be paid to subtle presentations such as anorexia, new urinary incontinence, falls, fatigue, decreased mental status, and impaired functional capacity. All can be early manifestations of an evolving pneumonia.

The physical findings seen in pneumonia such as rales, sonorous rhonchi, and consolidation appear to be similar in NHAP compared with the noninstitutionalized elderly. One note of caution: Functional atelectasis (crackles heard upon deep inspiration) can be seen in the elderly with a poor cough reflex and may mimic the crackles of pneumonia.

Diagnosis

Establishing the diagnosis of pneumonia in the nursing home setting is difficult at best. There have been few published multicenter studies that have addressed an approach to the evaluation of these pneumonias. Establishing a correct diagnosis is frustrating in the nursing home setting because the chest radiograph and laboratory are not on site, physician availability is not immediate, and aspiration is known to be common.

Two pieces of information should be obtained immediately when pneumonia is suspected. First are the vital signs. When the respiratory rate and pulse rate are increased greater than 25 breaths per minute and 100 beats per minute, respectively, without other explanation (combined with any respiratory symptoms), the suspicion of pneumonia should be great.

Second, oximetry is of great value. Kaye demonstrated that in the setting of infection, a decrease in the oxygen saturation from baseline of greater than 3% or a single saturation below 94% should suggest pneumonia (Kaye et al 2002). He further found that if these findings were not present, the diagnosis of pneumonia was unlikely.

Sputum analysis is problematic, first in obtaining a specimen and second in its interpretation. Fifty percent to 70% of residents of a long-term care facility are unable to produce sputum specimens adequate for analysis. When sputum is obtained, the physician must interpret the findings in light of known oropharyngeal colonization and the possibility of aspiration.

Because the clinical and laboratory findings are inconsistent in the elderly with pneumonia, it is particularly important to obtain a chest radiograph. In the nursing home setting, this is often performed by a mobile unit, a portable one-view film, making it less than desirable for diagnosis. Furthermore, when dehydrated, these patients may not manifest an infiltrate early in the disease course. With hydration, however, the infiltrate will become more apparent.

Finally, laboratory information may be nonspecific. The leukocyte count in this group may be low, normal, or elevated, and add little to the diagnosis. In the end, as most often in medicine, the diagnosis is based on a strong clinical suspicion.

Treatment

When planning therapy for NHAP, three questions must be addressed. First, does the patient have a chemical aspiration pneumonia or a bacterial pneumonia? Second, what is the most appropriate site of care for this patient: nursing home or hospital? Third, if the pneuomonia is bacterial, what antibiotic should be used?

With the high incidence of aspiration seen in the nursing home setting, it is often difficult to differentiate a chemical pneumonitis not requiring antibiotic therapy from a true bacterial process because both are associated with similar signs, symptoms, and radiographic findings. In a study of 195 episodes of suspected pneumonia by aspiration, Mylotte found that only 43 (21%) proved to be bacterial in origin (Mylotte et al 2003). Naughton and Mylotte (2000) recommended no use of antibiotics with a negative chest x-ray. If a patient has suspected or documented aspiration, he or she can be observed for 24 hours for the development of signs and symptoms of pneumonia. If these signs and symptoms occur, secondary bacterial infection should be suspected and antibiotics administered. However, the authors concluded that even in the presence of symptoms antibiotic treatment is probably not needed in patients with a negative x-ray.

The second important decision is whether the site of care should be a nursing home or a hospital. Extensive study has not been done on the process physicians should use when trying to make this decision, and no guidelines on the issue have been published. Many local factors play a role in this decision including laboratory, chest x-ray, physician, and support staff availability. One proposed strategy was observing the respiratory rate, which, if under 40 per minute, indicated mild-to-moderate pneumonia that could be treated in the nursing home, whereas a respiratory rate over 40 per minute indicated severe pneumonia requiring hospitalization. Several recent studies have demonstrated that the majority (63-78%) of patients with NHAP were treated without transfer to acute care. While the CAP guidelines would suggest hospitalization for most elderly patients, studies have shown that acute in-hospital care does not improve survival.

Specific antibiotic selection for NHAP has been poorly defined. Optimal antibiotic therapy should neither miss an important pathogen nor provide coverage that is too broad. Because of the common problem of obtaining sputum in the nursing home patient, therapy is most often empiric. Also, aspiration needs to be considered.

The CAP guidelines of both the Infectious Disease Society of America and the American Thoracic Society acknowledge that NHAP should be given special consideration. However, only the Canadian Infectious Disease guidelines propose specific antibiotic recommendations for NHAP. Oral quinolones are the preferred regimen, and amoxicillin-clavulanate plus a macrolide is the second choice. If the patient is hospitalized for the pneumonia, the recommendation is a quinolone as monotherapy and a second- or third-generation cephalosporin plus a macrolide as the next choice. The community standard for duration of therapy is 7-10 days. Pneumococcal resistance to antibiotics (especially penicillin and macrolides) also occurs in the elderly.

Outcome

The mortality from NHAP treated in the nursing home ranges from 6-28% compared with 20-40% in the hospitalized individual. This may represent selection with the more severely ill being hospitalized. The most important determinant for the outcome from NHAP is the patient's functional status, both for short- and long-term mortality. Underlying illness and age do not appear to play a significant role in the outcome.

Prevention

The patient living in a nursing home is at risk for NHAP not only because of advanced age and underlying illness but also because of confinement in an environment that promotes the spread of communicable disease. Prevention is therefore of paramount importance and is multifaceted. Beneficial measures include good general hygiene and nutrition, avoidance of medication that decreases mentation, minimizing aspiration, and nursing staff compliance with infection-control procedures. In addition, these individuals should be vaccinated for influenza and *S. pneumoniae* based on CDC guidelines. Finally, employees and patients should be screened for tuberculosis and appropriate preventive therapy administered when indicated.

Summary

NHAP represents a significant problem, from the cost of treatment to mortality and morbidity. NHAP differs from CAP and HAP in terms of its diagnosis and treatment. The diagnosis of pneumonia in the nursing home setting is highly problematic, requiring a high index of suspicion. Special considerations regarding treatment include distinguishing chemical pneumonitis from bacterial pneumonia, determining whether the patient can be treated in the nursing home setting or needs to be moved to an acute care facility, and choosing an antibiotic for these patients, in whom sputum analysis is often difficult. Despite these special features of NHAP, there are few specific guidelines addressing them. With the aging of the population, the need for nursing home care can only increase, and with it the need for optimal care and management.

BIBLIOGRAPHY AND SUGGESTED READING

Cunha BA. Pneumonia in the elderly. Clin Microbiol Infect. 2001;7:581-8. *State-of-the-art review.*

Feldman C. Pneumonia in the elderly. Med Clin North Am. 2001;85:1441-59. *Discusses changes in lung function and immunosenescence with aging as predisposing factors for pneumonia in the elderly.*

Janssens JP, Krause KH. Pneumonia in the very old. Lancet Infect Dis. 2004;4:112-24. *Extensive review and bibliography of all aspects of pneumonia in the elderly.*

Kaye KS, Stalam M, Shershen WE, et al. Utility of pulse oximetry in diagnosing pneumonia in nursing home residents. Am J Med Sci. 2002;324:237-42. *Describes use of noninvasive oxygen monitoring, citing the applications of pulse oximetry.*

Mandell LA, Marrie TJ, Grossman RF, et al. Canadian guidelines for the initial management of community-acquired pneumonia: an evidence-based update by the Canadian Infectious Disease Society and the Canadian Thoracic Society. Clin

Infect Dis. 2000;31:383-421. *Commonly used guidelines in Canada that may be appropriate for use in the United States.*

Marrie TJ. Pneumonia in the long-term-care facility. Infect Control Hosp Epidemiol. 2002;23:159-64. *Comprehensive review of NHAP.*

Mylotte J, Goodnough S, Naughton BJ. Pneumonia versus aspiration pneumonitis in nursing home residents: diagnosis and management. J Am Geriatr Soc. 2003;51:17-23. *Addresses the common problem of aspiration and its etiology.*

Naughton B, Mylotte J. Treatment guideline for nursing home–acquired pneumonia based on community practice. J Am Geriatr Soc. 2000;48:82-8. *Commonly used guidelines for practitioners who work in nursing homes.*

7 Tuberculosis and Other Mycobacterial Disease

The mycobacteria are a unique group of bacilli that are responsible for a variety of pulmonary and extrapulmonary infections, with a particular propensity to involve the elderly.

The mycobacteria evolved as organisms of the soil. To survive in extremes of temperature, wide swings in hydration, and periods of nutritional deprivation, they have thick waxy coats. This elaborate cell wall determines several traits that shape the transmission, pathogenesis, and treatment of mycobacterial infections: 1) they are not significantly influenced by humoral immunity but are controlled by the cellular immune system; 2) they replicate slowly, meaning that the time from infection to overt disease is prolonged and that therapy (which is bactericidal only during replication) must be prolonged; 3) their ability to resist dehydration facilitates airborne transmission; 4) they are resistant to many disinfectants; and 5) traditional antibiotics have limited efficacy against them.

Tuberculosis

Tuberculosis (TB) (caused by *Mycobacterium tuberculosis*) has been receding in incidence in the United States over the past decade due to increased clinical awareness, the effectiveness of directly observed therapy in halting transmission, and selective preventive therapy (now called "treatment of latent infection"). However, case rates remain relatively high in the elderly populations of all racial groups. This is the result of two factors: 1) the elderly lived in periods when TB was more prevalent and are therefore more likely to harbor latent infection; and 2) with the aging process there is predictable waning of immune competency, "immunosenescence," which increases the risk of reactivation.

Pulmonary disease is the most common form of TB, but the elderly experience an assortment of extrapulmonary (XP) disease as well. Approximately 25% of disease in the elderly involves sites outside the lung; a small portion have simultaneous pulmonary and XP-TB. The most common sites and forms of disease outside the lungs in the elderly include renal, osseous (spinal, hip and knee), and miliary.

Diagnosis

Important clinical pearls relating to TB in the elderly include the following:

- Although the majority of patients complain of feeling feverish, the absence of objective fever cannot exclude active TB, even extensive disease.
- As many as 25-50% of elderly patients with TB do not have a significant response to the tuberculin skin test (TST) or PPD.
- Up to half of those with sputum culture–positive pulmonary TB have negative sputum smears.
- In almost all cases it is appropriate to begin therapy on the presumption of a diagnosis of TB (e.g., do not wait for positive cultures if the clinical profile strongly suggests TB and no alternative diagnosis is evident).
- An elderly person who is recently infected (e.g., with a positive TST after exposure) is at extremely high risk for rapid progression to active disease, comparable with that for an infant. Classically, pulmonary TB involves the upper lobes with a predilection for the apical-posterior segments. However, clinicians should be aware that up to one third of elderly patients have lower zone or atypical radiographic presentations.

The "booster effect" with serial tuberculin skin testing (TST) was recognized in USPHS (U.S. Public Health Service) studies: it was observed that a higher percentage than anticipated became "new" reactors to the second annual TST. This was more common in the older subjects in the survey. It was inferred that the first TST placement did not elicit a positive reaction, but reawakened or boosted the cells responsible for delayed-type hypersensitivity to the TST. Thus, some patients appeared to have been recently infected when, in fact, they had merely been boosted. To avoid confusion, it has been advocated that, for any individual or group that is to be followed with serial TSTs (health care workers, medical or nursing students, employees at correctional facilities or nursing homes), initial two-step testing be performed. In this model, if the subject does not react to TST #1, a second TST is administered 1-4 weeks later. If the patient reacts to TST #2, the inference is that (s)he was boosted rather than infected during the interval. Clinically, this puts the individual in the category of having had remote infection rather than the higher-risk category of recent infection. Recently infected normal subjects have a 5-7% risk of developing active TB within 2 years, making them strong candidates for treatment of latent infection (TLTI), whereas an individual with no risk factors and remote TB infection may have only a 0.03-0.1% annual risk of TB, lessening the indication for TLTI. Although boosting is more common in older subjects, it occurs even in those in their 20s. Hence it is generally prudent to do two-step initial testing on all subjects for whom serial TSTs are planned. It should be noted that persons who had BCG vaccinations in childhood are at high risk for boosting. To be deemed a significant increase in reactivity, the size of the TST reaction should increase by 10 mm or more in induration.

Treatment

The medical management of active TB consists of the use of multiple drugs, which, in combination, enhance the efficacy of therapy, shorten the duration of disease, and prevent acquired drug resistance. Current guidelines of the American Thoracic Society (ATS) and CDC endorse the regimens described in Table 7-1 for the treatment of TB. The most important drug is rifampin (RIF); it is the keystone to shortened duration of therapy. Given *in vitro* susceptibility to and tolerance of RIF, it is possible to concoct a predictably effective regimen. Isoniazid (INH) is an important but not essential component of modern regimens; however, it entails a relatively higher risk of hepatitis among elderly patients (up to 3-5% in persons aged 65-85). Pyrazinamide (PZA) is used primarily to reduce treatment to 6 months. Ethambutol (EMB) has been used as a fourth drug in initial therapy due to the potential risk of further acquired resistance if the patient has primary drug resistance.

Among the elderly, PZA may result in disruptive GI distress, arthralgias, and a modest risk of hepatitis. Because shortened treatment is not of premier importance in older patients (they are at low risk of absconding from treatment], it is reasonable to omit PZA and employ a more benign regimen that would take 9 months to effect a cure. If one elects to omit PZA from initial therapy, it is appropriate to use EMB until *in vitro* susceptibility to RIF and INH is confirmed. If EMB is just used for the initial 2 months and renal

Table 7-1. Recommended Regimens for the Treatment of Tuberculosis (American Thoracic Society/Centers for Disease Control and Prevention)

I. 6-month Regimens

Initial Phase (2 months)	Continuation Phase (4 months)	
A. INH 300 mg daily	INH 300 mg daily or 900 mg twice-weekly	
RIF 600 mg daily	RIF 600 mg daily or 600 mg twice-weekly	
PZA 20-25 mg/kg daily		
EMB 15 mg/kg daily		
B. INH 600 mg thrice-weekly	INH 600 mg thrice-weekly	
RIF 600 mg thrice-weekly	RIF 600 mg thrice-weekly	
PZA 30-35 mg/kg thrice-weekly		
EMB 30-35 mg/kg thrice-weekly		

Initial Phase (2 wks)	Secondary Phase (6 wks)	Continuation Phase (18 Wks)
C. INH 300 mg daily	INH 900 mg twice-weekly	INH 900 mg twice-weekly
RIF 600 mg daily	RIF 600 mg twice-weekly	RIF 600 mg twice-weekly
PZA 20-25 mg/kg daily	PZA 25-35 mg/kg twice weekly	
EMB 15 mg/kg daily		EMB 35 mg/kg twice weekly

II. 9-Month Regimens

Initial Phase (2 months)	Continuation Phase (7 months)
INH 300 mg daily	INH 300 mg daily
RIF 600 mg daily	RIF 600 mg daily
EMB 15 mg/kg daily	

COMMENTARY: Regimen C is the most widely employed directly-observed therapy regimen in the U.S. Involving only 58 to 62 doses, it makes supervised treatment easier. In the first 2 weeks, treatment may be given 5 days per week (Monday–Friday) for convenience. The 2003 Guidelines also include rifapentine regimens that are not included here.

function is normal, visual acuity monitoring is not necessary. Whichever regimen is chosen, it is of vital importance to ensure that the drugs are given on a reliable basis: *directly-observed therapy* by a health professional has been standard procedure in many jurisdictions in the United States.

The question of multidrug-resistant TB or MDR-TB was a prominent issue in the 1990s. However, MDR-TB has receded overall in the United States (the current rate is less than 1%), and it is less prevalent in the elderly who likely contracted their infections before drug resistance became commonplace. However, all isolates of TB should be sent for *in vitro* susceptibility testing.

Prevention

For much of the world, vaccination has been the major element of protection against TB. Unfortunately, the vaccine, BCG (bacille Calmette-Guérin, a live attenuated strain of *M. bovis*, an organism closely related to TB), generally has failed to curtail tuberculosis in the adult and elderly populations. Although there have been reports indicating up to 80% protection, including in adults, all of these trials were done in the 1930-1950 era. All studies done since then have failed to demonstrate efficacy.

Based on skepticism about the protection afforded by BCG, U.S. authorities have employed "preventive therapy" or, as recently re-titled, "treatment of latent tuberculosis infection" as their central strategy. Epidemiologic studies have consistently shown that the majority of TB cases in the U.S. emerge from those who were infected remotely in time; thus, the strategy was developed of giving isoniazid (INH) to those thought to harbor latent infection. Latent infection was determined usually by significant reactivity to the tuberculin skin test (TST) or PPD ("purified protein derivative"). However, for some persons thought to be infected by virtue of exposure and at relatively great risk of progressing to active disease, treatment could be initiated despite failure to react to the TST. Examples include infants and persons with AIDS or other immunosuppressed states.

New guidelines for the treatment of latent infection were published in 2000. They involved these central elements:

- "Targeted tuberculin testing" is recommended; that is, we should only administer a TST if we intend to give preventive therapy when the test is positive.
- Instead of the 6- and 12-month durations for INH regimens, 9 months was recommended for all indications.
- Rather than biochemical monitoring for those at high risk for hepatitis, symptomatic surveillance was endorsed.
- For the first time, three alternative regimens were presented in addition to 9 months of INH: (*a*) 6 months of INH is an acceptable but not primary option; (*b*) 4 months of rifampin (RIF) was considered a secondary option except for persons with HIV/AIDS, for whom the fear of acquired rifamycin resistance made this unacceptable; and (*c*) a novel regimen of RIF and pyrazinamide (PZA) for 2 months daily or 3 months twice weekly was given a high rating, especially for persons with HIV/AIDS. Unfortunately, early experience with the RIF-PZA regimen resulted in unexpectedly high rates of morbidity (symptomatic hepatitis) and mortality (roughly 1 patient per 1000 started on this regimen in a CDC trial developed fatal hepatitis). Hence, the CDC and ATS have withdrawn this regimen from use.

Although the 2000 guidelines endorsed symptomatic monitoring for INH-related hepatitis, this may not be optimal in elderly persons with impaired cognition or communication ability. For instance, if treatment of latent infection is indicated for an outbreak in a nursing home, it might be suitable to monitor liver chemistries on a monthly basis in addition to symptomatic surveillance. Another option, given the relatively high risk for INH-related hepatitis in the elderly, would be to use RIF. RIF has a lesser risk of hepatitis and requires only 4 months for completion, but care must be taken regarding the potentially harmful drug interactions associated with RIF (see the *Physicians' Desk Reference* for more information).

Clinicians caring for the elderly must be aware of one recently identified risk factor for reactivation of TB: the use of tumor necrosis factor (TNF) modifying or inhibiting agents such as infliximab (Remicade) or etanercept (Enbrel). Given to patients with severe rheumatoid arthritis or inflammatory bowel disease, these agents have been associated with rapid development of severe, potentially fatal TB and other mycobacterial infections.

Environmental (Non-Tuberculous) Mycobacteria

Unlike TB, which is spread exclusively by human-to-human transmission, environmental mycobacteria (EM) are acquired from water, soil, or other sources in our natural or indoor environments.

In the first 75 years of the 20th century, human disease from EM was relatively uncommon (the estimated annual incidence in the United States circa 1980 was about 1 case per 100,000 population) and typically occurred in men whose lungs were damaged by cigarette smoking or inorganic dust exposure. However, over the past three decades there appears to be an emerging epidemic of lung disease caused by *Mycobacterium avium* complex (a cluster of strains of *M. avium* or *M. intracellulare*, referred to as MAC) and a rapidly growing mycobacterial species, *M. abscessus* or *M. chelonae*. While seemingly most prevalent in the southeastern United States, cases are now being seen in all 50 states and in Canada.

Much of this modern epidemic involves middle-aged to elderly, slender, white females, the majority of whom do not have readily identifiable risk factors such as smoking. And, unlike the males with COPD who typically had upper lobe cavitary disease similar to classic TB, these women most frequently have bronchiectasis. Even more intriguing, these women often have thoracic anomalies including narrow anterior-posterior diameter (with or without pectus excavatum), scoliosis, and/or mitral valve prolapse.

Diagnosis

The typical clinical presentation of such patients includes recurrent or chronically escalating cough, variably productive of purulent phlegm. Some patients experience insidious malaise and/or fatigue. Chest x-rays typically demonstrate bilateral amorphous features, although peri-cardiac shadowing with effacement of the heart borders suggests involvement of the RML and/or lingula.

If infection with EM is suspected, CT scanning and sputum collection for AFB are the fundamental diagnostic measures. When the patient cannot produce sputum, induction with hypertonic saline is the first step. If the symptoms persist and no sputum can be obtained, bronchoscopy is indicated to isolate mycobacteria or other potential pathogens such as *Pseudomonas aeruginosa*. The simultaneous recovery of gram-negative rod (GNR) species, such as *Pseudomonas, Alcaligenes*, and *Stenotrophomonas, and* EM is not rare. In some cases, one might consider treating for the GNR infection (usually 2 weeks of intravenous antibiotics) before initiating therapy for EM (which typically involves lengthier and more complex therapy).

In patients with bronchiectasis associated with EM, the regions most frequently and severely involved are the right-middle lobe and/or lingular segments of the left upper lobe. The diagnosis is made by demonstration on computed tomography (CT) scanning of bronchiectasis and centrilobular nodules along with recovery of the EM from sputum or bronchial lavage (for those unable to produce sputum).

Treatment

Management of patients with bronchiectasis associated with EM consists of a combination of antimicrobial therapy and bronchial hygiene.° For some patients in whom symptoms are modest and/or ill-defined, a 2-month therapeutic trial may be appropriate. In selected cases, surgical resection may be undertaken.

°The criteria for the diagnosis and treatment of EM lung disease are complex. The 1997 Guidelines of the American Thoracic Society for Non-tuberculous Mycobacterial Disease were well intended but overly complex and rather impractical; they are being re-written and are not referenced in this chapter. Based on considerable experience at the National Jewish Medical and Research Center, revised recommendations are delineated in the EM chapter of Gorbach's *Infectious Diseases*, 2nd ed; Philadelphia: Lippincott Williams & Wilkins; 2003.

The usual regimen for MAC entails a macrolide (AZI or CLARI), a rifamycin (RIF or RBU) and ethambutol (EMB). Clarithromycin (CLARI) is modestly more active than azithromycin (AZI) but generally results in more GI upset and dysgeusia. The meds may be given daily, but recent experience suggests that regimens of 3 times per week (Mon-Wed-Fri) are comparable in efficacy to daily regimens, are less expensive, and result in fewer side effects.

For rapidly growing mycobacteria, such as *M. chelonae* or *M. abscessus*, a 2- or 3-drug regimen is usually effective. *M. chelonae* is generally resistant to cefoxitin but has variable susceptibility to imipenem, amikacin, and clarithromycin. *M. abscessus* is usually susceptible to cefoxitin as well as amikacin and imipenem. Cures are rarely achieved with lung disease that is caused by rapidly growing mycobacteria; hence, we generally think in terms of suppressing the disease, similar to the model of *Pseudomonas* infection in patients with cystic fibrosis. Given the complexity of managing such infections, a full discussion of this topic is beyond the scope of this chapter (see Iseman and DeGroote 2003).

Bronchial hygiene consists of mechanical mucus clearance and inhaled therapy. Various devices may be employed to impart mechanical energy to the airways to mobilize tenacious secretions. Respiratory therapists can instruct patients in the use of such devices as the Acapella Valve, Flutter Valve, or PepValve, which may significantly enhance mucus clearance. The Thera-Vest has been used extensively in patients with cystic fibrosis; however, it may prove useful in other varieties of bronchiectasis. For patients with chronically inflamed and congested airways, inhalation of beta-agonists, anticholinergic bronchodilators, and/or steroids may enhance mucus clearance, reduce cough, and improve airflow. For those with particularly tenacious secretions, agents that loosen or break down secretions, such as N-acetylcysteine (Muco-myst) or hypertonic (3%) saline, may be beneficial.

The prognosis with treatment is less well studied than for TB. Unlike TB, in which enduring cures are expected with reliable therapy and drug-susceptible strains, the outcome of treatment of EM lung diseases is far less predictable. Although the great majority of EM patients show symptomatic, radiographic, and bacteriologic improvement with appropriate therapy, failure to become culture negative, relapses following cessation of therapy, and/or recrudescence secondary to exogenous reinfection (sometimes with EM species other than the original pathogen) are common among EM patients.

Surgery may be helpful by removing badly damaged lung units, particularly RML or lingula. However, such surgery is complicated due to inflammatory obliteration of anatomical landmarks and should be undertaken only by experienced thoracic surgeons.

BIBLIOGRAPHY AND SUGGESTED READING

I. TUBERCULOSIS

American Thoracic Society. Targeted tuberculin testing and treatment of latent tuberculosis infection. Am J Respir Crit Care Med. 2000;161:S221-S247. *Recommendations of the ATS and Centers for Disease Control identifying suitable candidates for skin testing and regimen options for preventive therapy. Note that despite an "expert" panel and evidence-based recommendations, this document unfortunately advocated an unacceptably toxic regimen, rifampin and pyrazinamide.*

Blumberg HM, Leonard MK Jr, Jasmer RM. Update on the treatment of tuberculosis and latent tuberculosis infection. JAMA. 2005;293:2776-84. *Excellent, concise review of the treatment of tuberculosis and latent tuberculosis infection.*

Centers for Disease Control. Targeted tuberculin testing and treatment of latent tuberculosis infection. MMWR. 2000;49:1-54 (No. RR-6).

Centers for Disease Control and Prevention (CDC), American Thoracic Society. Update: adverse event data and revised American Thoracic Society/CDC recommendations against the use of rifampin and pyrazinamide for treatment of latent tuberculosis infection-United States, 2003. MMWR. 2003;52:278-82. *ATS and CDC acknowledge that the RIF-PZA regimen entails too much risk of serious hepatitis and death to be recommended under any circumstances.*

Iseman MD. A Clinician's Guide to Tuberculosis. Philadelphia: Lippincott Williams & Wilkins; 2000. *Clinically oriented monograph that covers in detail the diagnosis, treatment and prevention of TB, including in the elderly.*

Menzies D, Dion MJ, Rabinovitch B, et al. Treatment completion and costs of a randomized trial of rifampin for 4 months versus isoniazid for 9 months. Am J Respir Crit Care Med. 2004;170:445-9. *Shows that, despite increased costs for the drug, RIF, the 4-month regimen of RIF was associated with higher completion rates, lesser morbidity, and overall reduced costs versus 9 months of INH.*

Wallis RS, Broder MS, Wong JY, et al. Granulomatous infectious diseases associated with tumor necrosis factor antagonists. Clin Infect Dis. 2004;38:1261-5. *Indicates that the use of tumor necrosis factor (TNF) modifying agents such as infliximab (Remicade) or etanercept (Enbrel) is associated with considerable risk of serious, even life-threatening infections due to TB or EM.*

II. ENVIRONMENTAL MYCOBACTERIA

Field SK, Fisher D, Cowie RL. Mycobacterium avium complex pulmonary disease in patients without HIV infection. Chest. 2004;126:566-81. *Covers MAC lung disease from a different aspect than the present chapter; suggests that defects in the interferon-gamma system increase the risk for MAC in elderly females.*

Iseman MD. Bronchiectasis. In: Mason B, Broaddus VC, Murray JF, Nadel JA, eds. Murray and Nadel's Textbook of Respiratory Medicine, 4th ed. Philadelphia: WB Saunders; 2005. *Addresses the etiology, risk factors, diagnosis, and management of the diverse forms of bronchiectasis with or without associated EM infection.*

Iseman MD, DeGroote M. Environmental mycobacterial (EM) infections. In: Gorbach SL, Bartlett JG, Blacklow NR, eds. Infectious Diseases, 3rd ed. Philadelphia: Lippincott Williams & Wilkins; 2003. *Addresses in detail the epidemiology, risk factors, diagnosis, and management of pulmonary and extrapulmonary disease due to EM.*

8 Venous Thromboembolism

enous thromboembolism (VTE) is manifested clinically by deep vein thrombosis (DVT) and pulmonary embolism (PE). Deep vein thrombosis, usually of the lower extremity, nearly always precedes PE. The risk of VTE increases greatly after age 50. In addition to age, major acquired risk factors are trauma, immobilization, and surgery. Other acquired risk factors are cancer and estrogen use in oral contraceptives and hormone replacement therapy (Table 8-1). The anti-estrogen tamoxifen also increases the risk of VTE. Individuals with inherited conditions that increase risk (thrombophilia) usually present before age 40, although it is not unusual to see the first episode of VTE in a patient with factor V Leiden appear after total hip replacement at age 65. The disease most often occurs in hospitalized patients, particularly those with cancer or following surgical procedures, but VTE also occurs sporadically in the community. In both settings, multiple risk factors are usually present.

Etiology

The triad of venous stasis, vessel wall injury, and instrinsic blood abnormalities (Virchow's triad) has been known for more than 150 years. Venous stasis (bedrest, immobilization, or paralysis) and vessel wall injury (surgery or trauma) are typically self-evident. Blood abnormalities (the third contributor) have been more thoroughly understood only in recent years with the

Table 8-1 Risk Factors for Venous Thromboembolism

Acquired	Inherited
• Age > 50	• Factor V Leiden
• Surgery	• Prothrombin gene mutation (G20210A)
• Trauma	• Antithrombin deficiency
• Immobility	• Protein C deficiency
• Cancer	• Protein S deficiency
• Estrogens, exogenous	• Elevated factors VIII or XI
• APAS	• MTHFR abnormalities

APAS = antiphospholipid antibody syndrome; MTHFR = methyltetrahydrofolate reductase.

indentification of multiple acquired and inherited conditions that lead to VTE (see Table 8-1).

Diagnosis

Diagnosis of VTE requires a high index of suspicion in anyone with unexplained dyspnea (PE) or leg swelling or pain (DVT). The diagnosis is particularly difficult in a geriatric population because PE can mimic a lingering pneumonia or congestive heart failure. It is important to remember that the great majority (97%) of patients with PE will have one or more symptoms or signs: dyspnea, pleuritic pain, and a respiratory rate greater than 20 per minute.

Spiral chest CT scanning with contrast has become increasingly accepted as the initial test of choice for diagnosing PE. The test is highly specific (>90%) but has an overall sensitivity of about 80% because it misses small PE in sub-segmental or smaller pulmonary arteries. To achieve acceptable sensitivity, spiral chest CT should be combined with a leg study such as duplex ultrasound or a venous phase leg CT from the same contrast injection used for the spiral chest CT. When both the spiral chest CT and a leg study are used, VTE is detected with greater than 90% sensitivity. When both tests are negative, it is acceptable to withhold anticoagulation unless the clinical suspicion of VTE continues to be high. In this circumstance, further testing is warranted with contrast venography, V/Q lung scans, or pulmonary angiography depending on the circumstances. In outpatients with low or moderate suspicion of VTE, a negative or normal serum D-dimer measurement is sufficient to withhold anticoagulation. Measurement of D-dimer is much less useful in the hospital because most inpatients have elevated D-dimer levels.

Treatment

Important elements of treatment of VTE are effective anticoagulation and early mobilization. LMWH is a good choice for initial therapy because it has a predictable anticoagulant effect and allows early hospital discharge or even home therapy in selected patients. LMWH products are dosed on body weight. No change in dose is necessary in the elderly. It is important to start warfarin on day 1 and overlap warfarin and the heparin product for at least 5 days, also confirming that the INR is in the target range of 2.0-3.0 before heparin is stopped. Shortening the course of unfractionated heparin or LMWH by starting warfarin on day 1 of VTE treatment is useful to minimize the risk of HIT. Whereas warfarin at 5-10 mg daily is often a suitable starting dose in younger patients, patients over age 65 and those weighing less than 40 kg should usually be started on a dose of 2-3 mg. These patients also often can be maintained on lower doses as well. The duration of anticoagulation should be tailored to assessment of both recurrence risk and bleeding risk (Table 8-2). Decisions about duration of anticoagulation should be made in conjunction with the patient's wishes and should include consideration of both the risk of bleeding and the risk of recurrence. Maintaining the INR in the target range of 2.0-3.0 minimizes recurrence risk without significantly increasing bleeding risks and is preferred over an INR range of 1.5-2.0 for long-term treatment of VTE. A frequently overlooked therapeutic intervention in patients with DVT is the use of elastic support hose. A well-fitted pair of below-knee elastic support hose (30-40 mm Hg at the

Table 8-2 Recommendations for Duration of Anticoagulation

Condition	Duration
1st event, transient risk factor	3-6 months
1st event, idiopathic VTE*	At least 6 months
1st event, with thrombophilia, cancer** or APAS	12 months to lifetime
Recurrent event	12 months to lifetime

*Idiopathic VTE is VTE that occurs without a known risk factor. It is also called primary VTE.

**For cancer patients with VTE, anticoagulation with treatment dose LMWH is recommended for 3-6 months. At that point the decision should be made whether to continue with LMWH or switch to warfarin (INR 2-3).

ankle) worn for 2 years has been shown to reduce the long-term rate of post-phlebitic thrombotic syndrome by 50% (Prandoni et al 2004).

Treatment in Special Populations

Heparin-induced thrombocytopenia (HIT) occurs when antibodies to a heparin-platelet factor 4 complex induce platelet activation and consumption. The extreme example of the clinical consequence of HIT is arterial or venous thrombosis (HITTS). Stroke, myocardial infarction, VTE, and limb or bowel ischemia can occur. HIT should be suspected any time the platelet count falls below 100,000/μL or otherwise falls by 50% compared with baseline. Fortunately, HIT is rare, occurring in less than 1% of patients who receive heparin. Orthopedic surgery patients, who receive heparin for longer than 7 days, and cardiac surgery patients, who receive heparin in interrupted intervals, are at highest risk. The syndrome usually appears between the fifth and tenth day of therapy, although it can occur earlier in patients who have had recent exposure to heparin. It can also appear later or even after therapy has stopped, particularly in patients receiving LMWH. When HIT is suspected, heparin should be stopped and therapy begun with a parenteral direct thrombin inhibitor, either argatroban or lepirudin (Refludan). Warfarin should not be used at this point; if it has already been started, it should be stopped and its effect reversed with vitamin K. This is because warfarin can block the fibrinolytic process and cause what is termed "warfarin necrosis." HIT is divided into two types: one that is reversible, and one that is a rare type with fatal implications. Consultation with a hematologist is advised in some cases of HIT.

Antiphospholipid antibody syndrome (APAS) occurs spontaneously and in association with a number of medical conditions, notably connective tissue diseases. The phenomenon was first recognized as the lupus anticoagulant syndrome, which is named for its association with systemic lupus erythematosus (SLE), although a circulating anticoagulant of this type can occur in the absence of SLE. The syndrome predisposes to both arterial and venous thrombosis. When VTE occurs in conjunction with APAS, treatment is similar to that given to other patients with VTE. Some authorities also recommend adding aspirin 81 mg daily because of the increased risk of arterial thrombosis associated with APAS.

In patients with renal failure, special considerations with regard to anticoagulants should be addressed. All the LMWHs and fondaparinux (Arixtra) are cleared renally, and these drugs can accumulate in plasma in patients with creatinine clearances below 30 mL/min. This consideration is particularly important in the frail elderly who may have decreased renal function despite a serum creatinine at the upper end of the normal range. Recently, guidelines have been issued to clarify the use of enoxaparin in patients with significant renal insufficiency (creatinine >1.8) as recommended in the package insert and PDR.

Cancer patients with VTE are at higher risk of both recurrence and death than other patients with VTE. Because of improved treatment and longer survival, cancer patients account for an increasing proportion of those with VTE. VTE can occur before cancer is evident, at the time of diagnosis of cancer, and at any point in the clinical course of patients with known cancer. VTE is particularly likely to occur during intensive chemotherapy and as a complication of cancer surgery. For years clinicians have been aware of so-called "warfarin failure" in patients with VTE and cancer (i.e., the tendency to suffer recurrent VTE despite an INR between 2.0 and 3.0). Recent clinical trials have shown that long-term LMWH in a treatment dose reduces the recurrence rate of VTE in cancer patients by 50% compared with wafarin (INR 2-3). The new therapeutic recommendation for treatment of cancer patients with VTE is LMWH in a treatment dose for 3-6 months. At that point the clinician has the option of continuing the LMWH or switching to warfarin (INR 2-3).

Newer Therapies

Fondaparinux (Arixtra)

Fondaparinux is a small (molecular weight 1726 daltons), synthetic, indirect factor Xa inhibitor. It is a parenteral agent given subcutaneously once daily. It acts by binding to antithrombin and facilitating antithrombin's inhibition of factor Xa. In this regard it is similar to LMWH, but its small size and synthetic nature make it a different class of drug. Fondaparinux does not require monitoring or dose adjustment in patients who have normal to moderately impaired renal function. The incidence of HIT appears to be negligible with fondaparinux, and the drug has actually been used to treat patients with HIT. Fondaparinux currently has indications for prevention and treatment of VTE. It has been shown to be particularly effective in preventing VTE after hip fracture surgery when given for 1 month following surgery.

Direct Thrombin Inhibitors

Direct thrombin inhibitors bind directly to the active site of thrombin without need of the cofactor, antithrombin. The first of these experimental agents, ximelagatran, has been withdrawn from the market because of liver toxicity. However, several other direct thrombin inhibitors are currently under study. Ximelagatran is a pro-drug given twice daily in a fixed dose and does not require anticoagulation monitoring or dose adjustment. The drug is rapidly hydrolyzed to the active agent, melagatran. Melagatran is cleared renally and dose adjustments are probably necessary in patients with severe renal impairment (creatinine clearance less than 30 mL/min). The drug's onset of action occurs within 1 hour, and consequently it would have theoretically been useful for both acute and chronic treatment of thrombotic diseases.

Prevention

Prevention of VTE is especially important in older patients who are undergoing surgery or are hospitalized for a medical condition. Surgical patients at highest risk include those undergoing orthopedic procedures on the lower extremity and those undergoing cancer surgery. Medical patients at high risk include those with heart or respiratory failure, stroke, cancer, and serious infections such as pneumonia. Table 8-3 gives recommended prophylactic measures in patients according to risk group.

The syndrome of "economy class VTE" seems to be precipitated by immobilization and dehydration associated with long airplane flights. Risk appears to increase greatly when a flight exceeds 5 hours. On long flights, older travelers should get out of their seats and walk around the cabin every 2 hours. Wearing a pair of surgical support hose during the flight is also a good idea. Travelers with a prior history of VTE or who are otherwise at increased risk should probably receive a subcutaneous injection of low-molecular-weight heparin (LMWH), fondaparinux (Arixtra), or unfractionated heparin, before boarding the flight. The prophylactic benefit of aspirin in this setting is uncertain but is likely to be small.

Table 8-3 Recommendations for Prophylaxis of Venous Thromboembolism

Indication	Recommendation
Medically ill	UFH, LMWH, or fondaparinux
General surgery	UFH or LMWH
Neurosurgery	IPC or LMWH
Cardiovascular surgery	UFH or LMWH
Cancer surgery	LMWH or UFH
Orthopedic surgery	Fondaparinux, LMWH, or warfarin
Spinal cord injury	LMWH, UFH, or warfarin

UFH = unfractionated heparin; LMWH = low molecular weight heparin; IPC = intermittent pneumatic compression.

BIBLIOGRAPHY AND SUGGESTED READING

Eriksson BI, Lassen MR, Gent M, et al. Duration of prophylaxis against venous thromboembolism with fondaparinux after hip fracture surgery. Arch Intern Med. 2003;163;1337-42. *Compared to fondaparinux given for 1 week after hip fracture surgery, extending prophylaxis to 4 weeks reduced both venographic DVT and clinical recurrence.*

Francis CW, Davidson BL, Berkowitz SD, et al. Ximelagatran versus warfarin for the prevention of venous thromboembolism after total knee arthroplasty. Ann Intern Med. 2002;137:648-55. *Ximelagatran started after total knee replacement was at least as effective as warfarin (INR2-3) in preventing venographic DVT.*

Hyers TM. Management of venous thromboembolism: past, present and future. Arch Intern Med. 2003;163:759-68. *Overview of progress in treatment and prevention of VTE, including description of new anticoagulants.*

Lee AYY, Levine MN, Baker RI, et al. Low-molecular-weight heparin versus coumarin for the prevention of recurrent venous thromboembolism in patients with cancer. N Engl J Med. 2003;349:146-53. *In cancer patients with VTE, dalteparin continued for 6 months cut VTE recurrence rate in half compared with warfarin at an INR 2-3.*

Prandoni P, Lensing AWA, Prins MH, et al. Below-knee elastic compression stockings to prevent the post-thrombotic syndrome—a randomized, controlled trial. Ann Intern Med. 2004;141:249-56. *Well-fitted, below-the-knee surgical support hose worn for 2 years after DVT reduced the incidence of post-thrombotic syndrome by 50% over a 5-year follow-up.*

9 Interstitial Lung Disease

nterstitial lung disease (ILD) refers to a heterogeneous group of pulmonary disorders characterized by diffuse parenchymal involvement. The prevalence of these diseases in the elderly varies with each specific disorder. In the elderly patient, trying to identify a potential causative factor or etiologic association is often the initial priority. Of the interstitial lung diseases that do not have an identifiable cause, idiopathic pulmonary fibrosis is particularly associated with middle-aged to elderly patients, typically between 50 and 70 years of age.

The various disorders producing ILD frequently have similar clinical, physiologic, and roentgenographic manifestations. Often there may be both interstitial and alveolar involvement so the term *interstitial lung disease* can be misleading. A more descriptive but infrequently used term is *diffuse lung disease*. The purpose of this chapter is to focus on the diseases that primarily affect the interstitium (the area between the alveoli and capillaries) but at times may have an alveolar component. It remains important to exclude other disorders such as congestive heart failure, chronic aspiration, adverse drug reactions, and acute and chronic infections, which may appear similar to ILD. This chapter focuses on the entity of ILD, not the numerous potential causes of interstitial abnormalities.

Diagnosis

Clinical Presentation

Patients with ILD generally complain of dyspnea (especially with exertion) and cough. The cough is usually dry and non-productive and varies from the mild irritating variety to disabling paroxysms associated with gagging, chest wall discomfort, and even near syncope. Chest pain as an isolated symptom rarely occurs. With severe ILD and pulmonary hypertension, patients may develop chest pain indistinguishable from angina. Pleuritic chest pain is not associated with ILD, and other causes must be explored. Chest wall and musculoskeletal discomfort occur from chronic coughing. Hemoptysis is not associated with typical idiopathic ILD; however, it can occur with pulmonary vasculitis and alveolar hemorrhage syndromes. Symptoms may be insidious in the elderly. At times a family member may be the first to notice a change in exercise tolerance, a gradual reduction in activity, or a persistent cough. When questioned, the patient almost always admits to shortness of breath with activity and frequently attributes this to aging, deconditioning, or a persistent "chest cold." Dyspnea on exertion is the most common complaint of patients with ILD. Unfortunately, this is true of most patients with any form of chronic heart or lung disease. The chronic production of mucus, especially in large amounts, is not a part of ILD and is more suggestive of chronic bronchitis or bronchiectasis.

Asymptomatic patients with ILD may be diagnosed because of an abnormal chest x-ray or computed tomographic scan (see "Radiographic Imaging" section). With the more frequent use of electron beam computed tomography to screen for coronary artery disease, more incidental cases of ILD are being discovered. With the increased use of screening spirometry, primary care physicians are finding patients with both obstructive (COPD patients) and restrictive (ILD patients) abnormalities. The typical restrictive pattern that characterizes the ILDs is a reduction in lung volumes, particularly total lung (TLC), accompanied by a decrease in both the FEV_1 (forced expiratory volume at 1 second) and FVC (forced vital capacity) with a normal or increased FEV_1 to FVC ratio (>75%).

History

The patient history gives direction to further evaluation. In the symptomatic patient (e.g., with dyspnea) the physician should establish: 1) How long have symptoms been present? 2) Are symptoms stable, escalating, or decreasing? and 3) Are other active medical conditions present? An acute onset suggests an active inflammatory etiology that usually responds well to therapy (Table 9-1). Environmental history should review exposure to pets (especially birds), humidifiers, swamp coolers, molds, recurrent home water damage, or organic dusts. Occupational history can reveal exposure to asbestos, silica, beryllium, and coal dust, as well as inhaled gases and chemicals. In older patients, especially those with neuromuscular disease or previous cerebrovascular

Table 9-1 Duration of Interstitial Lung Disease Before Diagnosis As Related to Etiology*

Acute (days to few weeks)

• Bronchiolitis obliterans with organizing pneumonia (cryptogenic organizing pneumonia)

• Extrinsic allergic alveolitis (hypersensitivity pneumonitis)

• Acute idiopathic interstitial pneumonia (Hamman-Rich syndrome)

• Some drug reactions (e.g., amiodarone, nitrofurantoin)

• Radiation pneumonitis

Subacute (weeks to months)

• Connective tissue disease

• Alveolar hemorrhage syndromes

• Sarcoidosis

• Drug reaction (cytotoxic agents)

• Bronchiolitis obliterans with organizing pneumonia

• Radiation pneumonitis

Chronic (months to years)

• Idiopathic pulmonary fibrosis

• Silicosis

• Asbestosis

• Coal workers' pneumoconiosis

• Sarcoidosis

• Chronic aspiration

*There may be overlap, with many causes of ILD presenting in both subacute and chronic forms.

accidents, chronic aspiration may lead to a form of ILD. A complete list of current medications may reveal drugs capable of producing lung disease. Amiodarone, nitrofurantoin, and cytotoxic chemotherapeutic agents are most commonly involved. Previous radiation therapy to a part or majority of the thorax may result in radiation pneumonitis and/or fibrosis. The combination of radiation and chemotherapy may increase the risk of pulmonary toxicity.

Physical Examination

The classic finding in ILD is the presence of coarse rales or crackles, sometimes termed "Velcro rales." In early or limited disease they are found primarily at the lung bases, but they are more diffuse with more extensive parenchymal involvement. They will not clear with coughing and deep breathing. Loud crackles may be present with minimal abnormalities on the chest x-ray. With chronic idiopathic ILD (idiopathic pulmonary fibrosis or IPF), the crackles persist and do not decrease even with therapy that results in other clinical improvement. With the more acute and subacute presentations, the crackles diminish with clinical improvement. Patients with extensive interstitial abnormalities on chest x-ray and few or no crackles on exam usually have old granulomatous disease (e.g., sarcoid) or pneumoconiosis (e.g., silicosis or asbestosis) and not IPF.

Clubbing occurs primarily in IPF (which corresponds to a histopathologic appearance called "usual interstitial pneumonia") and rarely in other forms of ILD. The base of the nail bed is spongy and the angle of the nail bed changes from a concave shape to one that is convex. Clubbing is generally associated with more advanced disease and greater physiologic impairment.

With advanced ILD, patients develop pulmonary hypertension, cor pulmonale, and refractory hypoxemia that accelerates the pulmonary hypertension. Supraventricular arrhythmias are common; the pulmonic component of the second heart sound is accentuated (increased P2) and, clinically, the patient becomes intolerant of any activity.

Laboratory Studies

Initial studies should include a complete blood count, biochemical survey to evaluate renal and hepatic function, erythrocyte sedimentation rate, urinalysis, and electrocardiogram. There are several serologic studies available that may be helpful in identifying various disorders that result in interstitial lung disease (Table 9-2).

Radiographic Imaging

Although the chest x-ray remains the simplest and most informative study available, patients with early ILD may have a normal CXR. In typical ILD the parenchyma has increased interstitial markings frequently described as reticular (linear) or reticulonodular. An alveolar or acinar component may be present when nodular densities become more confluent. The predominant pattern, however, is interstitial involvement. This is typical of idiopathic pulmonary fibrosis, sarcoidosis, silicosis, asbestosis, and other pneumoconioses. When the pattern becomes more alveolar (soft homogeneous shadowing) with or without air bronchograms, alveolar filling diseases such as bacterial pneumonia, congestive heart failure, bronchioloalveolar cell carcinoma, and alveolar hemorrhage must be considered.

Table 9-2 Laboratory Studies Used in Interstitial Lung Disease

Test	Diagnosis*
Antinuclear antibody (ANA)	Systemic lupus erythematosus
Anti-JO antibody	Scleroderma
Rheumatoid factor (RF)	Rheumatoid arthritis
Antineutrophil cytoplasmic antibody (ANCA)	Wegener's granulomatosis
Antiglomerular basement membrane antibodies	Goodpasture's syndrome
Serum precipitating antibodies (hypersensitivity pneumonitis panel)	Hypersensitivity pneumonitis
Serum immune complexes	Idiopathic pulmonary fibrosis, lymphocytic interstitial pneumonia, systemic vasculitis
Angiotensin converting enzyme (ACE)	Sarcoidosis
RBC casts in urine	Systemic vasculitis, connective tissue disease

*Test is not always specific for but is consistent with the listed diagnosis. Negative serum test does not always exclude the listed diagnosis.

Enlarged hilar structures can be representative of hilar adenopathy, enlarged pulmonary arteries, or masses. The finding of bilateral, symmetrical hilar adenopathy with or without associated ILD is classic for sarcoidosis. With unilateral or asymmetric hilar adenopathy, lymphoma must be excluded. With unilateral hilar enlargement and ipsilateral interstitial infiltrates, carcinoma with lymphangitic spread is likely. When ILD and enlarged pulmonary arteries are simultaneously present, the disease is in an advanced stage and the patient also suffers from pulmonary hypertension.

Computed tomography with contrast is usually necessary to accurately distinguish hilar adenopathy from enlarged pulmonary arteries. Assessing the pattern and location of diffuse parenchymal abnormalities can be helpful. Hypersensitivity pneumonitis, silicosis, and sarcoidosis tend to have upper lobe predominance, while idiopathic pulmonary fibrosis, asbestosis, and ILD associated with connective tissue disease tend to involve the lower lobes.

Computed Tomography

CT scans of the chest have revolutionized the approach to pulmonary disease. Standard helical (spiral) CT can be done with or without contrast. The high-resolution technique (HRCT) is ideal for evaluating the lung parenchyma. No contrast is used in HRCT, which images representative portions of the lung in 1-cm intervals with 1-mm slices. If contrast is needed to evaluate vascular and hilar structures, a second CT scan should be performed after the HRCT and contrast can then be injected. In early cases of ILD the chest x-ray may be normal and only by using HRCT can ILD be detected. As with the chest x-ray, characterizing the parenchymal abnormalities helps to establish the diagnosis. Nodular infiltrates are commonly found in sarcoidosis, bronchiolitis, silicosis, and pneumoconiosis. Interlobular septal thickening is more consistent with idiopathic pulmonary fibrosis (IPF), ILD secondary to connective tissue disease, lymphangitic carcinomatosis, and asbestosis (Table 9-3).

The HRCT pattern of IPF commonly shows patchy bibasilar, peripheral, and subpleural reticular abnormalities. There is variability in the amount of

Table 9-3 Common Appearance of Parenchymal Abnormalities on Imaging Studies in Diffuse Lung Disease

Appearance	Disease
Nodules	• Sarcoidosis • Military tuberculosis • Coal workers' pneumoconiosis • Eosinophilic granuloma (Langerhans cell histiocytosis) • Metastatic disease • Silicosis
Interlobular septal thickening	• Idiopathic pulmonary fibrosis • Connective tissue disease • Asbestosis • Sarcoidosis • Lymphangitic carcinomatosis
Alveolar opacification/Ground-glass shadowing	• Desquamative interstitial pneumonia • Drug reactions • Alveolar proteinosis • Acute bacterial pneumonia • Bronchiolitis obliterans with organizing pneumonia (cryptogenic organizing pneumonia) • Pulmonary edema • Bronchioloalveolar cell carcinoma • Hypersensitivity pneumonitis
Cystic changes	• Emphysema • Lymphangioleiomyomatosis • Idiopathic pulmonary fibrosis • Connective tissue disease • Asbestosis • Eosinophilic granuloma (Langerhans cell histiocytosis)
Pleural involvement	• Asbestosis • Amiodarone reaction • Connective tissue disease

Modified from Albert RK, Spiro SG, Jett JR, eds. Comprehensive Respiratory Medicine. London: Mosby; 1999.

alveolar (ground-glass) opacity present. In areas with severe involvement, honeycombing and traction bronchiectasis are present.

With HRCT, much more precise anatomic localization is possible and the relationship between the lung and pleural and mediastinal structures is well defined. Well-trained radiologists with a special interest in HRCT of the chest can accurately diagnose the etiology of ILD in a high percentage of cases. In institutions where such specialization is not available, the accurate diagnosis of ILD by HRCT is variable and many times requires a tissue diagnosis.

Pulmonary Function Testing

Complete pulmonary function studies including spirometry, lung volumes, diffusing capacity, and resting and exercise oximetry (6-minute walk) should be performed. If oximetry is normal, room air arterial blood gases can be obtained to determine whether the alveolar-arterial oxygen difference is abnormal (increased). Most of the diseases causing ILD will result in a restrictive physiologic pattern. Typically the forced expiratory volume in 1 second (FEV_1) and forced vital capacity (FVC) are reduced (<80% of predicted) and the FEV_1/FVC ratio is normal or increased (>75%). Lung volumes are also reduced, with total lung capacity, residual volume, and functional residual capacity frequently being less than 80% of predicted. The single breath carbon monoxide diffusing capacity (DLCO) is also reduced, even when corrected for reduced lung volumes. If studies of lung compliance (volume/pressure) are performed, the lungs are usually stiff and noncompliant. Thus, these patients require greater pleural pressure swings (more negative pleural pressure on inspiration) to generate adequate tidal volumes, resulting in a higher work of breathing. Patients who respond to therapy generally have improvement in pulmonary function and the distance they can cover in a 6-minute walk. Those with progressive disease, especially those with idiopathic pulmonary fibrosis, demonstrate continued loss of pulmonary function.

Biopsy

Lung biopsy is not necessarily required to make a clinical diagnosis of ILD, but only a biopsy can establish a specific histologic pattern. In older patients with a clinical picture, an x-ray pattern, and a suspected clinical diagnosis suggesting a potential response to corticosteroids (e.g., bronchiolitis obliterans, NSIP, DIP), a therapeutic trial may be appropriate. For patients in whom the differential diagnosis is broad, or if there is presumed infection not responding to antibiotic therapy, bronchoscopy with bronchoalveolar lavage and transbronchial biopsy may be helpful. In many situations, going directly to video-assisted thoracoscopic lung biopsy (VATS) is indicated.

Fiberoptic bronchoscopy (FOB) has its limitations. If infection is likely, especially *Pneumocystis jiroveci* (formerly *carinii*), then FOB with broncho-alveolar lavage is indicated. If sarcoidosis or lymphangitic carcinomatosis is a likely etiology, then FOB with transbronchial biopsy is appropriate.

Because of the limited tissue sample from transbronchial biopsy, the VATS approach is far superior to establish the cause of ILD in all situations other than those listed above. In institutions where VATS is performed on a routine basis, both morbidity and mortality are low and the benefits from having an accurate tissue diagnosis outweigh the risks, especially when patients continue to deteriorate. Lung biopsies should be from several sites and should sample both normal and abnormal lung tissue. The final benefit to VATS biopsy is to categorize the specific type of interstitial process that is occurring in patients with idiopathic interstitial lung disease (e.g., usual interstitial pneumonia vs. nonspecific interstitial pneumonitis) because emerging therapies are different.

Idiopathic Interstitial Pneumonia and Idiopathic Pulmonary Fibrosis

When other causes of ILD have been eliminated, the diagnosis of idiopathic interstitial pneumonia is made. For years physicians have attempted to classify this heterogeneous group of illnesses, which may have similar clinical presentations, laboratory values, and radiographic findings. Finally, in 2000 the American Thoracic Society (ATS) and the European Respiratory Society published guidelines regarding the diagnosis and treatment of idiopathic pulmonary fibrosis (IPF), the most common of the idiopathic interstitial pneumonias. Because the natural history of disease and response to therapy of the various histologic subtypes of idiopathic interstitial pneumonias can vary widely, an attempt to provide a specific tissue diagnosis is usually indicated. Patients with IPF have the histologic pattern of usual interstitial pneumonia (UIP). Other potential pathologic patterns on biopsies of patients with idiopathic interstitial pneumonia ILD similar to IPF include: nonspecific interstitial pneumonia (NSIP), desquamative interstitial pneumonia (DIP), respiratory bronchiolitis-associated interstitial lung disease (RBILD), acute interstitial pneumonia (AIP), and bronchiolitis obliterans organizing pneumonia (BOOP). These diagnoses are considered separate entities and represent different diseases from IPF. At times more than one histological pattern may be present, complicating therapeutic decisions.

At present there are no proven therapies for IPF. IPF is a progressive disease that usually affects individuals 50 years of age and older. Males are affected more commonly than females. For years IPF was thought to be the result of chronic inflammation that resulted in parenchymal fibrosis. The assumption that interruption of the inflammatory cascade early in the illness would prevent irreversible tissue injury seemed logical. For years the mainstay of treatment for IPF was corticosteroids and cytotoxic therapy. It is now clear that current anti-inflammatory therapy for IPF provides little or no benefit. Thus new hypotheses and therapies are needed.

Researchers are beginning to focus more on the fibrotic process and less on the inflammatory cascade. The histological hallmarks of IPF are fibroblastic foci, which appear as nodules of spindle cells arranged in linear fashion against pale staining extracellular matrices. Adjacent alveoli may be spared, and there is no necrosis or substantial inflammation. It seems more likely that IPF results from a combination of sequential acute lung injury and exaggerated wound-healing (excessive fibroblast replication and matrix deposition) that culminates in pulmonary fibrosis. Many factors may modify this fibrotic response, including genetic background, environmental triggers such as cigarette smoking or respiratory toxins, and viral infections.

Treatment

Anti-Inflammatory Agents

Systemic corticosteroid administration with or without immunosuppressive therapy remains the treatment of choice for ILD associated with connective tissue disease, hypersensitivity pneumonitis, BOOP, NSIP, and sarcoidosis. Generally these diseases respond more favorably to treatment than IPF. Earlier studies found response rates of 10-40% in patients with IPF who were treated with systemic corticosteroids and/or cytotoxic agents. However in these studies, other types of interstitial pneumonias (e.g., NSIP) were not excluded. In more recent studies limited to patients with IPF, the administration of corticosteroids and cytotoxic drugs was of no benefit. While many of the other types of idiopathic interstitial pneumonia, such as NSIP, DIP, BOOP, and RBILD, respond well to corticosteroids alone, sometimes the addition of cytotoxic drugs such as cyclophosphamide (Cytoxan) or azathioprine (Imuran) is required.

When a tissue diagnosis is not available to establish a diagnosis in the elderly, it may be difficult to distinguish between IPF and other interstitial pneumonias. In this situation, many pulmonary physicians will empirically treat with prednisone for a limited period (3-6 weeks) and observe for symptomatic relief (reduction in cough or dyspnea) and physiologic improvement. If the patient does not improve, azathioprine (Imuran) or cyclophosphamide (Cytoxan) can be added. If there is no response after 8-12 weeks of therapy, treatment should be discontinued. In these situations therapy must be individualized because side effects or adverse drug reactions may require an earlier discontinuation of medications.

Antifibrotic Agents and Immune Modulators

Interferon gamma, a Th1 cytokine, down-regulates the expression of transforming growth factor beta-1, a mediator strongly implicated in fibroblastic proliferation and collagen deposition.

In 1999 a preliminary study evaluating interferon gamma-1ß therapy (Actimmune) in patients with IPF not responsive to corticosteroids and immunosuppressive agents suggested improved pulmonary function and gas exchange after 3 months of therapy. A placebo-controlled trial followed and, during a median of 58 weeks, interferon gamma-1ß did not significantly prevent progression of disease or deterioration in pulmonary function, nor did it improve quality of life. However, there was a suggestion of improved survival in the treatment group (Raghu et al 2004). A third, more comprehensive study is underway.

Currently interferon gamma-1ß is available for treatment of IPF. The patient receives 200 μg subcutaneously three times per week. The most common side effects are flu-like symptoms, including headache, fever, and chills. The decision to use the drug is on an individual basis and depends on a diagnosis of IPF (UIP), age, ability to receive home injections, and insurance coverage for the drug. (The cost is approximately $50,000 per year.) Therapy is continued indefinitely as long as the patient shows either clinical improvement or stabilization. Most pulmonary physicians favor treating only patients with biopsy-proven disease because of the extremely poor prognosis and only a suggestion that survival is improved. Because lung transplantation is limited to patients with end-stage lung disease who are younger than 65 years of age, it is not a therapeutic consideration in the elderly.

Summary

Although a great deal of attention has been given to idiopathic interstitial pneumonias, the clinician must keep in mind that these are relatively uncommon diagnoses compared with other illnesses that can cause diffuse pulmonary infiltrates. When an elderly patient presents with cough, shortness of breath, hypoxemia, and increased interstitial markings on chest x-ray, the clinician should first exclude: 1) congestive heart failure (systolic or diastolic); 2) atypical pneumonia; 3) recurrent, chronic aspiration; and 4) drug-induced lung disease (e.g., amiodarone). Once these are excluded, the quest for another diagnosis can begin.

BIBLIOGRAPHY AND SUGGESTED READING

Albert RK, Spiro SG, Jett JR, eds. Comprehensive Respiratory Medicine. London: Mosby; 1999. *Excellent reference text for overview of respiratory physiology and general discussion of ILD. The unique format and display of tables provide a refreshing change from the classic textbook approach.*

American Thoracic Society and European Respiratory Society Consensus Group. ATS guidelines. Idiopathic pulmonary fibrosis: diagnosis and treatment. Am J Respir Crit Care Med. 2000;161:646. *Important consensus statement that outlines the criteria for diagnosis of idiopathic pulmonary fibrosis. Description of the histologic patterns for other forms of idiopathic interstitial lung disease such as NSIP, RBILD, ALD, BOOP, and DIP is provided. An in-depth discussion of risk factors for IPF, diagnostic approaches, roentgenographic findings (CXR and HRCT), and treatment is also provided.*

Gross TJ, Hunninghake GW. Idiopathic pulmonary fibrosis. N Engl J Med. 2001;345: 517-25. *Review article discussing new concepts in the pathogenesis of idiopathic pulmonary fibrosis. Classic examples of lung biopsies, HRCT, and CXR are discussed. The therapy section looks at different potential therapies given the newer insights into the pathogenesis of IPF.*

Hunninghake GW, Lynch DA, Galvin Jr, et al. Radiologic findings are strongly associated with a pathologic diagnosis of usual interstitial pneumonia. Chest. 2003;124:1215-23. *This paper confirms other studies suggesting that well-trained radiologists can diagnose the type of ILD using high-resolution computed tomography. In this study of patients who presented with a clinical syndrome suggestive of IPF, HRCT findings of lower-lobe honeycombing and upper lobe irregular linear densities were usually found to confirm a pathologic diagnosis of UIP.*

Katzenstein AL, Myers JL. Idiopathic pulmonary fibrosis: clinical relevance of pathologic classification. Am J Respir Crit Care Med. 1998;157:1301-15. *State-of-the-art review that details the pathologic classification of ILD.*

Raghu G, Brown KK, Bradford WZ, et al, for the Idiopathic Pulmonary Fibrosis Study Group. A placebo-controlled trial of interferon gamma 1-ß in patients with idiopathic pulmonary fibrosis. N Engl J Med. 2004;350:125-33. *Multinational trial in which 330 patients unresponsive to corticosteroid therapy were randomized to receive interferon gamma 1-ß or placebo.*

Schwarz MI, King TE Jr. Approach to the evaluation and diagnosis of interstitial lung disease. In: King TE Jr, Schwarz MI, eds. Interstitial Lung Disease, 4th ed. Ontario, Canada: BC Decker; 2003. *Excellent chapter in a classic textbook on ILD. The text is superb throughout, with many tables and diagrams to illustrate important points.*`

10 Congestive Heart Failure

ongestive heart failure (CHF) is predominantly a disease of the elderly. The prevalence and incidence of heart failure increase with age, rising from a prevalence of 3% in patients older than 50 years to approximately 1 out of 10 patients older than 70 years. Patients over the age of 70 years account for 50% of all cases of CHF. As the baby boomers age and new technology improves the survival of heart disease, CHF will become pandemic in the early 21st century.

The prognosis of CHF is directly related to the cause, and the degree, of left ventricular (LV) dysfunction and the presence of its symptoms. The diagnosis of idiopathic cardiomyopathy usually has a better prognosis than that of ischemic cardiomyopathy. Patients with NYHA class I-II heart failure (Table 10-1) have a 5-10% annual mortality, NYHA class III an annual mortality of 20%, and NYHA class IV an annual mortality of 50% or greater. Heart failure is inexorably progressive and, during the decade following diagnosis, regardless of etiology, less than half of the patients survive. The mechanism

Table 10-1 New York Heart Association Classification System

Class I	No symptoms with ordinary activity: no limitation of physical activity
Class II	Symptoms with ordinary activity: mild limitation of physical activity
Class III	Symptoms with less than ordinary activity: marked limitation of physical activity
Class IV	Symptoms at rest: severe limitation of physical activity

Republished with permission from Criteria Committee, New York Heart Association. Diseases of the Heart and Blood Vessels: Nomenclature and Criteria for Diagnosis, 6th ed. Boston: Little, Brown; 1964.

of death is sudden cardiac death in 40% of patients, progressive heart failure in another 40%, and other causes in the remaining 20%.

Etiology

The etiologies of CHF are varied and include entities responsible for both systolic and diastolic CHF. The most frequently encountered LV systolic dysfunction diagnoses are ischemic, idiopathic, hypertensive, and alcohol-induced cardiomyopathy. However, a practicing physician may also see cardiomyopathies related to the peripartum period, obesity, hemochromatosis, myocarditis, AIDS, drugs (adriamycin or cocaine), and prolonged tachycardia (usually rapid atrial fibrillation).

Infections and anemia are probably the most common precipitating factors for CHF. Hypertension, once a more common cause of decompensated heart failure, is a significant contributor in the African-American population. Alcohol consumption is an often unrecognized and underestimated cause of cardiomyopathy and may account for up to 30% of all non-ischemic cardiomyopathy, independent of the amount of alcohol consumed. Rapid atrial fibrillation or flutter may cause a tachycardia-induced cardiomyopathy that usually normalizes after restoration of normal sinus rhythm. Certain drugs such as doxorubicin (adriamycin) may cause myocyte toxicity and cardiomyopathy in as many as 20% of patients receiving >700 mg/kg doxorubicin. Nonsteroidal anti-inflammatory drugs (NSAIDs), frequently prescribed to the elderly for arthritis relief, may alter prostaglandin-sensitive renal blood flow, leading to fluid retention and the exacerbation of heart failure. Glitazones (e.g., Actos and Avandia) are common hypoglycemic agents for adult-onset diabetes used frequently in the elderly population. However, they may precipitate heart failure by fluid retention and should be avoided in diabetic heart failure patients.

Diagnosis

The diagnosis of CHF is made by clinical and supporting laboratory criteria. In patients at risk of developing heart failure, such as those with prior myocardial infarction (MI), hypertension, or valvular heart disease, symptoms such as dyspnea on exertion, fatigue, or exertional intolerance may herald the development of heart failure. The cardinal elements of the history include the symptoms of congestion (orthopnea, paroxysmal nocturnal dyspnea [PND], edema) and symptoms of low cardiac output (fatigue and altered mental status). The physical exam should also be focused on establishing evidence of congestion or low cardiac output (CO). The presence of orthopnea,

		Congestion?	
		No	**Yes**
Low Perfusion?	**No**	Warm and dry PCWP normal, CI normal	Warm and wet PCWP elevated, CI normal
	Yes	Cold and dry PCWP low or normal, CI low	Cold and wet PCWP elevated, CI low

Signs of low perfusion	*Warm* and *cold* refer to skin temperature	**Signs of congestion**
• Narrow pulse pressure • Cool extremities • Obtundation • Vasodilator-related hypotension • Renal insufficiency	*Dry* and *wet* refer to presence or absence of lung crackles or edema	• Orthopnea • Jugular venous distention • Rales • S3 • Hepatojugular reflux • Ascites • Edema

Figure 10-1 Classification of patients with heart failure. (Adapted from Nohria A, Levine E, Arner SL. Management of heart failure. JAMA. 2002;287:628-40. Copyright ©2002, American Medical Association. All rights reserved.)

jugular venous distention (JVD), an S3, crackles (uncommon in CHF due to increased lymphatic drainage), ascites, hepatojugular reflux (HJR), hepato-megaly, and edema establishes the degree of congestion. A narrow pulse pressure, pulsus alternans, cool extremities, lethargy, and/or obtundation are the hallmarks of low cardiac output.

A brief bedside assessment can establish the diagnosis of CHF and clas-sify the hemodynamics necessary to guide appropriate therapy (Figure 10-1). Four categories readily describe CHF as adequately treated and compensat-ed (warm and dry), inadequately treated and decompensated (warm and wet, cold and wet), and finally, over-treated (cold and dry).

The laboratory evaluation of heart failure is helpful not only in deter-mining its severity, but also in establishing possible reversible causes and predicting prognosis. Minimal tests should include a basic metabolic panel with renal function, TSH, ECG, echocardiogram, ferritin, CXR, urinalysis, calcium, phosphate, CBC, and, if appropriate, an evaluation for underlying heart disease.

The finding of Q waves on an ECG may establish the presence of myocardial infarction and ischemic heart disease. Poor R wave progression is a frequent finding not only in ischemic heart disease but in non-ischemic diagnoses. A non-specific conduction defect or left bundle branch block (LBBB) is frequently seen in non-ischemic etiologies. Increased voltage and atrial enlargement may suggest underlying hypertensive heart disease, and tachycardia is usually indicative of significant decompensation.

A chest radiograph may show findings ranging from pulmonary venous hypertension to overt pulmonary edema, but may also show characteristics of a specific cardiac diagnosis such as rheumatic heart disease, cardiomegaly with an enlarged or hypertrophied LV, or a normal cardiac silhouette of diastolic dysfunction.

The level of B-type natriuretic peptide (BNP), a relatively new test, may establish the diagnosis of CHF if not clinically apparent, but is especially powerful in its negative predictive value to rule out dyspnea from a cardiac cause. The basic metabolic panel, including measure of renal function, is important, especially in assessing perfusion states and monitoring therapy such as renal angiotensin-aldosterone system (RAAS) inhibitors and diuretics. An abnormal TSH may be indicative of hypo- or hyperthyroidism, either of which can be responsible for heart failure. An abnormal ferritin may indicate hemochromatosis, an infiltrative disease that ultimately leads to dilated cardiomyopathy and heart failure.

Of all the laboratory studies for heart failure, an echocardiogram may be the most informative. It establishes the presence and severity of LV dysfunction, assesses global vs regional (ischemic) LV dysfunction, determines valvular function, excludes LV thrombus, and estimates LV filling pressures and pulmonary pressures.

Myocardial biopsy has a limited role but may be of benefit if infiltrative disease is suspected. A myocardial biopsy is no longer thought useful to direct therapy in suspected myocarditis, as treatment with immunosuppressive agents has shown no benefit.

A careful search for precipitating factors of heart failure should be undertaken to tailor therapy. Frequently, these precipitants manifest as acute occurrences that precipitously increase myocardial demand by placing an extra hemodynamic load on the heart. As mentioned earlier, infections and anemia are probably the most common acute precipitants, but it is imperative to exclude reversible ischemia in any patient with the established diagnosis of coronary artery disease (CAD) or at significant risk for ischemic heart disease. Hypertension should be adequately assessed and treated, especially in the African-American population. (Other important causes to search for are described earlier in the "Etiology" section.)

Treatment

The goals of heart failure management are three-fold: amelioration of symptoms, prevention or reversal of LV dysfunction, and prolongation of survival. The mainstays of management are non-pharmacologic therapies, pharmacologic therapies, and, finally, mechanical therapies.

Nonpharmacologic Therapy

The non-pharmacologic therapies are rooted primarily in diet and activity. Dietary restriction of salt is appropriate: patients with mild heart failure (NYHA class I-II) should consume a <3 g sodium diet, and patients with more advanced heart failure (NYHA II-IV) should consume a <2 g sodium diet. Fluid restriction is advisable, and patients should be limited to <2 liters/d, decreasing to <1.5 L/day when serum sodium falls below 125 mEq/L. Alcohol intake should be restricted to 1 drink per day or total abstinence in patients with alcoholic cardiomyopathy. Activity to prevent deconditioning is very important, and patients should be advised to exercise at least 5 days a week as tolerated. Walking is an excellent and well-tolerated activity. Elderly patients should be encouraged to walk initially 10 minutes a day and gradually increase in duration and speed until able to walk up to 30 minutes or more a day at a pace that causes mild breathlessness while conversing. Any type of isometric activity should be discouraged and avoided, including heavy weight lifting, although toning exercises with low weights and multiple repetitions are acceptable. A good rule of thumb is to lift no more than 20 pounds.

A formal cardiac rehabilitation or exercise program is appropriate for stable and motivated patients. Patients can return to work but should avoid heavy or sustained isometric activity and may have to limit their workday or other extracurricular activities. A scheduled nap time may prevent late-day fatigue. Sexual activity is usually well tolerated but may provoke uncomfortable dyspnea (such dyspnea often responds to pre-coital sublingual nitroglycerin). Patients prescribed the phosphodiesterase V inhibitors (Viagra, Levitra, Cialis, etc.) should be advised not to take concomitant sublingual nitroglycerin or alpha-blockers. The latter are often prescribed for benign prostatic hypertrophy, a common diagnosis in the elderly.

Pharmacologic Therapy

Although pharmacologic therapies have historically been prescribed for symptom relief, the greatest advances recently have been in the development of agents that prolong survival, prevent the progression of LV dysfunction (adverse remodeling), and reduce the need for hospitalization that accounts for the bulk of resource utilization. Approximately 50% of hospitalized patients discharged with the diagnosis of CHF are readmitted within 90 days. Table 10-2 outlines each class of drug/devices and their role in heart failure.

The management of heart failure is a continuum, from asymptomatic LV dysfunction to severe symptomatic heart failure. As the disease progresses, more heart failure agents are added rather than substituted and polypharmacy soon develops that creates many clinical challenges, especially in the elderly. Multiple co-morbidities, together with an aging circulation, may make the elderly patient intolerant of optimal doses of heart failure medications. Elderly patients frequently have a degree of autonomic dysfunction that aggravates the postural hypotension that accompanies vasodilator therapy. Vasodilator therapy may be further limited by the presence of cerebrovascular disease and the need to maintain an adequate systemic blood pressure for cerebral perfusion. The age-related decline in renal function of the elderly may lead to progressive renal insufficiency with diuretic and angiotensin-convering enzyme inhibitor (ACEI) therapy. Diastolic dysfunction is frequent in the elderly population and accounts for a significant proportion of heart failure in this age group. Diastolic dysfunction is very volume sensitive and may limit effective use of diuretic therapy (see "Diastolic Heart Failure" section later in this chapter).

Diuretics

Diuretics are used solely for symptomatic relief of congestion. A diuretic should be prescribed until the patient is euvolemic and then a determination made whether a maintenance dose is necessary versus symptom-driven dosing. If the patient becomes less responsive to increasing doses of a loop diuretic, a thiazide diuretic can be added 30 minutes prior to the loop diuretic to optimize the synergistic effect. The addition of a thiazide diuretic should be intermittent and symptom-driven, as tachyphylaxis may develop with long-term use. A caution to diuretic therapy is over-diuresis, which will stimulate the RAAS, clearly an unwanted effect of therapy in a heart failure patient. Over-diuresis can be detected by a metabolic panel demonstrating an elevation of the blood urea nitrogen (BUN) in a pre-renal pattern (BUN:creatinine > 20:1).

Table 10-2 Drug and Device Therapy for Systolic Heart Failure

Drug	Symptom reduction?	Mortality reduction?	Prevents progression?	Reduces hospital-ization?	Population targeted
Diuretics	Yes	No	No	Yes	Pulmonary congestion
ACE inhibitors	Yes	Yes	Yes	Yes	All
ARBs	Yes	Yes	Yes	Yes	ACE intolerant ? Triple Rx
Beta-blockers	Yes	Yes	Yes	Yes	NYHA II-IV ? All
Digoxin	Yes	No	No	Yes	AF or Sx after ACE/BB/diuretic
Spironolactone	Yes	Yes	Yes	Yes	NYHA III-IV
Calcium channel blockers (CCB)	Yes	No	No	No	HTN or angina
Nitrates + hydralazine	Yes	Yes	?	?	Intolerant ACE+ARB HTN/angina Pulmonary congestion
Anticoagulation	No	No	No	No	AF or LV thrombus
Antiarrhythmics	?	Trend (amiodarone)	No	?	EP selected patients
AICD	No	Yes	No	No	Post-MI LVEF < 30% +selected pts
Cardiac resynchronization	Yes	No	Yes	Yes	QRS > 130 ms LVEF < 35% NYHA III-IV

Angiotensin-Converting Enzyme Inhibitors

The ACEIs have been shown to improve symptoms, reduce mortality, and prevent hospitalizations in patients with heart failure. ACE inhibition is the first line of therapy for all patients with LV dysfunction, regardless of symptom status. Relative contraindications include hyperkalemia (K^+ > 5.5 mEq/L), renal insufficiency (creatinine >3.0 mg/dL), and hypotension (SBP <90 mm Hg). Hyperkalemia may respond to discontinuation of potassium supplements. Both hypotension and renal insufficiency are common, usually occur when the patient is volume-depleted from excessive diuresis, and usually respond to altering the diuretic dose. Other nephrotoxic drugs should be avoided, especially the NSAIDs. If the creatinine and BUN increase by less than 50%, the ACEIs can usually be continued, but if the rise in creatinine or BUN is greater than 50%, the dose of the ACEI should be adjusted downward by at least 50%. A continued rise in the creatinine or BUN to greater than 200% baseline should prompt discontinuation of the ACEI. If an ACEI is discontinued for either renal insufficiency or hyperkalemia, an angiotensin receptor blocker (ARB) should *not* be substituted, because the mechanism of action is similar.

There are two concerning side effects to ACEI therapy: cough and angioedema. The dry cough complicating an ACEI usually manifests by 2 weeks after onset of therapy and is often described as a persistent throat tickle in approximately 5-10% of patients on an ACEI. Unfortunately, the cough does not usually respond to switching to a different ACEI. The cough may take several days to weeks to resolve. An ARB is an attractive alternative (see below) and is infrequently associated with cough. An ACE-related cough should subside before initiating ARB therapy. Angioedema is usually insidious in onset and manifests, in most cases, within 2 weeks of therapy, although it may occur after months to years. Patients often complain that they have a fat lip or thick tongue or notice drooling. The presence of angioedema is an absolute contraindication for ACEI, and possibly also for an ARB.

Angiotensin Receptor Blockers

The role of ARBs has been controversial in the treatment of CHF. By blocking the angiotensin receptor, the ARBs more completely inhibit the RAAS. It is widely accepted that ARBs are an acceptable substitute for a patient intolerant to ACEI because of cough and possibly angioedema. Multiple randomized clinical trials have established a mortality and symptom benefit of ARBs as a substitute for ACEIs in the heart failure patient with systolic dysfunction. However, a subgroup analysis of the Val-HeFT trial showed a trend toward harm if the ARB valsartan was added to ACEI plus beta-blocker (BB) therapy. The CHARM study, a randomized, placebo-controlled trial designed to answer the question of triple therapy safety (Pfeffer et al 2003) showed: 1) the ARB candesartan reduced mortality in patients with heart failure; 2) the reduction in mortality was as robust as the reduction of mortality seen in some of the ACEI trials, suggesting that ARBs may possibly be used instead of an ACEI; 3) there was an incremental increase in mortality benefit with the addition of the ARB candesartan to existing ACEI + BB therapy; and 4) there was no mortality benefit with ARB therapy in patients

with preserved LV function (LV ejection fraction [LVEF] >40%), but hospitalizations were significantly reduced. The powerful findings of the
CHARM study, especially if confirmed by future studies, suggest that triple
therapy with ACEI+BB+ARB may become the new standard for the treatment of heart failure.

Beta-Adrenergic Blockers

Beta-adrenergic blockers (BBs), once considered contraindicated in heart
failure, are now first-line therapy for symptomatic heart failure (NYHA
II-IV) and impart a significant mortality benefit. Only three BBs
(carvedilol, metoprolol succinate [Toprol], and bisoprolol) have been
approved and should be used to the exclusion of other, possibly cheaper,
BBs until these latter agents have been shown beneficial. ACEI are usually initiated first, then BBs, unless in the post-MI or tachycardia patient
there is an indication for prompt administration of BBs. The BBs should
be started in patients with compensated heart failure who are euvolemic.
The dosing schedule should be slow, with an initial low dose and then
small dosage increases every 2-4 weeks as tolerated. There is often a
worsening of heart failure with the initiation of BBs. In these circumstances, as well as with other episodes of decompensation of heart failure,
more aggressive diuretic therapy and salt restriction with only a reduction
in BB dose may be all that is needed. It is not advisable to stop BBs once
initiated for heart failure due to the risk of clinical deterioration, even if
LV function normalizes and the patient is asymptomatic. If there is evidence of heart block, other chronotropic medications such as digoxin or
amiodarone should be adjusted or discontinued. Hypotension is a frequent side effect of BB therapy, more commonly if the patient is volume-
depleted from over-diuresis, and usually responds to dose decrease of
other heart failure medications such as diuretics or ACEIs or ARBs,
including staggering the dosing schedules.

Aldosterone Antagonists

Aldosterone antagonists have been shown to have both a symptom and mortality benefit in patients with advanced heart failure (NYHA II-IV and LVEF
<35%) and should be prescribed in these patients if the creatinine <2.0
mg/dL and K^+ <4.5 mEq/L (Pitt et al 1999). A daily dose of spironolactone
25 mg is sufficient. Potassium supplements should be reduced or withheld.
Eplerenone, a synthetic aldosterone inhibitor, has been shown to reduce
mortality in patients with heart failure following myocardial infarction and an
LVEF of <40%. Gynecomastia, often painful, is an unwanted side effect of
spironolactone but is rare with eplerenone.

Digoxin

Digitalis was the mainstay of symptomatic heart failure medication therapy until displaced by ACEI and BB therapy. Digoxin, the preferred agent, now plays a limited role and is usually reserved for: 1) patients still symptomatic after diuretic, ACEI, and BB therapy, especially if an S3 is present on exam; and 2) patients who have atrial fibrillation. No mortality benefit for digoxin has ever been established, but often heart failure will clinically worsen if digoxin therapy is withdrawn, although less so if the patient is on doses of diuretics and ACEI therapy that may be further adjusted to compensate for the withdrawal of digoxin. Digoxin toxicity is a clinical diagnosis. Digoxin efficacy has a poor correlation with serum levels, and digoxin dosing should *not* be titrated to serum levels. In elderly patients with normal renal function, a digoxin dose of 0.25 mg per day is usually well tolerated, but in elderly patients with renal insufficiency (creatinine >1.5 mg/dL), the dose should be halved to 0.125 mg per day. In elderly patients with significant renal insufficiency (creatinine >2.0 mg/dL), digoxin therapy is best avoided altogether.

Other Pharmacologic Agents

There are few randomized data concerning calcium channel blockers (CCB) in patients with heart failure. The dihydropyridine class drug amlodipine showed no symptom or mortality benefit in heart failure patients in the PRAISE study, although it did suggest a benefit in non-ischemic heart failure. Amlodipine (Norvasc) is often used as an adjunctive medication to control angina or hypertension in heart failure patients.

The first medications to show a mortality benefit in heart failure were hydralazine and nitrates in the VeHeFT trial. The medications were used in high doses, unlike usual practice; therefore, it is unclear if the mortality benefit would be achievable with more standard doses. The use of the combination regimen of nitrates and hydralazine is primarily reserved for those patients intolerant of ACEI and ARB due to renal insufficiency or hyperkalemia. Nitrates alone may be useful for symptomatic relief of pulmonary congestion, and hydralazine alone for patients who remain hypertensive despite BB, ACEI, and/or ARB therapy

Anti-Arrhythmic Therapy

Anti-arrhythmic therapy is a complex issue and is best decided by cardiology referral, preferably to an electrophysiologist. Half of the deaths in heart failure patients are due to sudden cardiac death, presumably arrhythmic. Patients with sustained ventricular tachycardia or survivors of cardiac arrest due to ventricular tachycardia/ventricular fibrillation (VT/VF) and other carefully selected patients with heart failure may enjoy increased survival with implantation of an automatic defibrillator (AICD) (Moss et al 2002). Amiodarone has been shown to be safe in patients with systolic LV dysfunction and may reduce the incidence of arrhythmic death with a trend toward increased survival in selected patients.

Mechanical Therapy

For the most part, mechanical therapy plays a limited role in the management of heart failure in the elderly population. In a subgroup of patients with symptomatic heart failure despite optimal therapy, LVEF <35%, and QRS duration >130 msec on EKG, cardiac resynchronization therapy (CRT) with bi-ventricular pacing may afford significant symptomatic relief. LV assist devices have historically been used as a bridge to transplantation but now are being studied for a possible expanded role of such supportive devices. The role of transplantation is quite limited in the elderly.

Other Treatment Considerations

The use of anticoagulation remains controversial in the management of heart failure patients. In the absence of compelling data to support its routine use in severe LV dysfunction (LVEF <35%), anticoagulation is generally recommended for patients with evidence of LV thrombus, atrial fibrillation, deep venous thrombosis (DVT), or thromboembolism (TBE), including pulmonary embolism (PE).

Intensive patient education programs and heart failure clinics with ancillary services such as social workers and home health nurses have reduced exacerbations and progression of heart failure, improved the quality of life, and significantly reduced (50%) hospitalizations for patients with heart failure.

Diastolic Heart Failure

Heart failure in patients with preserved LV systolic function (LVEF >40%) is a frequent finding in the elderly, accounting for up to 40% of patients. The most common presentation of heart failure with preserved systolic function is the elderly patient with hypertension and diabetes. In these patients, diastolic dysfunction from a stiff ventricle with abnormal ventricular relaxation and compliance, rather than decreased LV contractility, is responsible for the elevated cardiac pressures and pulmonary congestion. The impaired relaxation of the LV results in a markedly reduced LV end-diastolic volume that, despite a normal ejection fraction, is responsible for a lower stroke volume and cardiac output. The principal signs and symptoms are usually those of avid fluid retention. "Flash pulmonary edema" is not uncommon and is often precipitated by ischemia, renal artery stenosis, uncontrolled hypertension, dietary indiscretion, or medication non-compliance.

Despite the improved prognosis of diastolic heart failure compared with systolic failure, therapy can be frustrating. Diastolic dysfunction is highly volume sensitive, and very small increases in LV end-diastolic volume can translate into high pulmonary pressures and congestion. There is a very small window of volume tolerance, and the first-line therapy of diuretics may induce low cardiac output hypotension and renal insufficiency prior to the relief of congestion. There are no studies showing consistent benefit of drug therapy in diastolic heart failure, although the CHARM trial showed a symptom benefit with candesartan in reducing hospitalizations. The role of CCBs has been controversial regarding possible improved LV relaxation; furthermore, the use of CCBs is usually reserved for the treatment of hypertension. Management should be directed to diuretic therapy for congestion, tight control of hypertension, and control or elimination of tachycardia (which results in reduced diastolic fill time and lower stroke volume). Atrial fibrillation, frequent in the elderly, may present a special problem because it results in not only the loss of the atrial contribution to cardiac output but, possibly, in poorly controlled tachycardia. Aggressive attempts at maintaining sinus rhythm may be appropriate.

Right Heart Failure and Pulmonary Hypertension

Heart failure is frequently classified as left-sided, right-sided, or bi-ventricular. The most common cause of right heart failure is left heart failure. Occasionally, the practicing physician will encounter a patient who appears to have isolated right heart failure. A careful evaluation is important to rule out underlying left heart failure. Rales may be absent in biventricular failure as a result of enhanced pulmonary lymphatic drainage, and the major findings may be only those related to the systemic congestion of right heart failure. In this circumstance, treatment should be directed at management of the underlying LV failure. In contrast, if there is truly isolated right heart failure, the cause is almost always cor pulmonale. The most common cause of acute cor pulmonale is pulmonary embolus, but cor pulmonale is also frequently seen in chronic pulmonary embolus syndrome. The most frequent cause of chronic cor pulmonale is chronic hypoxemia. In the absence of a classic precipitating cause of pulmonary embolus such as DVT, a thorough search for hypercoagulability states or *in situ* pulmonary thrombosis should be initiated. Chronic anticoagulation and/or an inferior vena cava (IVC) interruption filter (temporary or permanent) are the therapies of choice. In those patients with chronic, recurrent pulmonary emboli in the proximal pulmonary artery bed and severe pulmonary hypertension unresponsive to classic anticoagulation therapy, pulmonary thromboendarterectomy may be beneficial in carefully selected patients.

Other causes of secondary pulmonary hypertension in the elderly include chronic obstructive pulmonary disease (the most common cause of hypoxia-induced pulmonary hypertension), interstitial lung disease, connective tissue disease (progressive systemic sclerosis, rheumatoid arthritis, or lupus), sleep apnea syndrome, obesity-hypoventilation syndrome, and kyphoscoliosis. Aggressive management of the underlying precipitating disease state, when available, and oxygen therapy for hypoxia-induced pulmonary hypertension remain the most important components of therapy. Phlebotomy may be necessary in patients with significant polycythemia. Despite the success of vasodilators such as epoprostenol, iloprost, bosentan, treprostinol, calcium channel blockers, and phosphodiesterase 5 (PDE5) inhibitors (sildenafil) in primary pulmonary hypertension (rare in the elderly) or pulmonary hypertension related to the scleroderma spectrum of diseases, these vasodilators have failed to produce sustained benefit in the treatment of secondary pulmonary hypertension. The use of vasodilators for treatment of secondary pulmonary hypertension therefore remains controversial and is the subject of on-going research. The routine use of warfarin has shown a morbidity and a mortality benefit in primary pulmonary hypertension (PPH), but its role has yet to be established in randomized clinical trials for the treatment of secondary pulmonary hypertension. Warfarin is indicated, however, in secondary pulmonary hypertension occurring in patients with a high risk of thromboembolism, such as those with prior pulmonary embolism or atrial fibrillation.

Summary

Heart failure and the co-morbidities that complicate its management are common in the elderly. With thoughtful attention to each patient's individualized needs, successful management plans can be established that will yield improved survival and quality of life for patients with heart failure.

BIBLIOGRAPHY AND SUGGESTED READING

Digitalis Investigation Group. The effect of digoxin on mortality and morbidity in patients with heart failure. N Engl J Med. 1997;336:525-33. *Excellent review of the oldest heart medication and its appropriate present day use in heart failure.*

Francis GS, Tang WHW. Heart failure due to systolic dysfunction. In: Crawford MH, DiMarco JP, Paulus WJ, eds. Cardiology, 2nd ed. Philadelphia: Mosby; 2004. *Readable and practical chapter on the nuts and bolts of treating heart failure.*

Heart Outcomes Prevention Evaluation (HOPE) Study Investigators. Effect of an angiotensin-converting inhibitor, ramipril, on cardiovascular events in high risk patients. N Engl J Med. 2000;342:145-53. *Adds to the previous studies establishing benefit of ACEI in the treatment of cardiovascular disease by showing a benefit in reduction of future cardiovascular events.*

Hunt SA, Baker DW, Chin MH, et al. ACC/AHA Guidelines for the Evaluation and Management of Chronic Heart Failure in the Adult: Executive Summary. Circulation. 2001;104:2996-3007. *Consensus opinion of how to apply evidence-based medicine to the bedside.*

Massie BM, Shah NB. Evolving trends in the epidemiology of heart failure: rationale for preventive strategies and comprehensive disease management. Am Heart J. 1997;133:703-12. *Excellent paper on the epidemiology of heart failure.*

Moss AJ, Zareba W, Hall WJ, et al. Prophylactic implantation of a defibrillator in patients with myocardial infarction and reduced ejection fraction. N Engl J Med. 2002;346:877-83. *Major study establishing the prophylactic use of AICD in the management of severe ischemic heart disease.*

Nohria A, Lewis E, Stevenson LW. Medical management of advanced heart failure. JAMA. 2002;287:628-40. *Excellent resource for the how's and why's of treating heart failure.*

Packer M, Bristow MR, Cohn JN, et al. The effect of carvedilol on morbidity and mortality in patients with chronic heart failure. N Engl J Med. 1996;334:1349-55. *Classic study establishing beta-blockers as first-line therapy for heart failure.*

Pfeffer MA, Swedberg K, Granger CB, et al. Effects of candesartan on mortality and morbidity in patients with chronic heart failure: the CHARM overall programme. Lancet. 2003;362:759-66. *Major study of the impact of ARB therapy in heart failure.*

Pitt B, Zannard F, Remme WJ, et al. The effects of spironolactone on morbidity and mortality in patients with severe heart failure. Randomized Aldactone Evaluation Study Investigators. N Engl J Med. 1999;341:709-17. *First study to show a mortality benefit of spironolactone treatment in advanced symptomatic heart failure.*

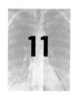

11 Asthma and Chronic Obstructive Pulmonary Disease

irway obstructive disease (asthma and chronic obstructive pulmonary disease [COPD]) is commonly encountered in the elderly patient. Approximately 10% of the population is believed to have COPD; another 10% to have asthma. Thus, 1 in every 5 patients seen by the primary care physician may have airway disease.

COPD has classically been taught to be a disease of the elderly, rarely being identified before the fifth decade of life. COPD is also found in younger individuals with alpha-1 antitrypsin deficiency, most commonly those who have the ZZ genotype.

Asthma, however, is considered by most of the lay public and by many physicians to be a pediatric disease. Therefore, the diagnosis of asthma tends to be overlooked in the elderly patient. Only recently has the medical community started to realize that asthma is nearly as common in the older adult as in the younger age group.

A compounding problem is the difficulty in differentiating between the two conditions, especially because asthma and COPD may co-exist in the same patient. Many patients with COPD respond to treatment more like asthmatics (and are often described as having "asthmatic bronchitis"), and many asthmatics who have never smoked develop irreversible chronic airway obstruction. Making distinctions between these diseases is often difficult, even for the experienced clinician, yet every effort should be made to do so because the approach to treatment may be different. Figure 11-1 demonstrates the overlapping of these disease processes; Table 11-1 lists the differential diagnosis.

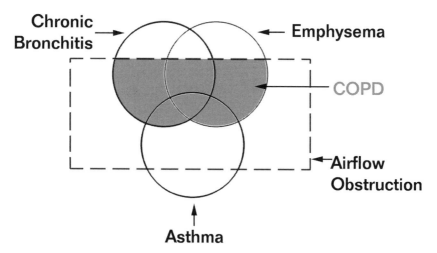

Figure 11-1 Overlapping of asthma and chronic obstructive pulmonary disease.

Table 11-1 Differentiating COPD and Asthma

COPD	Asthma
• Usually over age 40	• Usually under age 40
• Smoker	• Non-smoker
• Symptoms with exertion	• Symptoms anytime (often at night)
• Allergic history not prominent	• Allergic history prominent
• Bronchodilator response ($\Delta FEV_1 < 15\%$)	• Bronchodilator response ($\Delta FEV_1 > 25\%$)

Asthma

Prevalence

Little research has been done on the elderly with asthma. The true prevalence and incidence of asthma in this age group are difficult to establish because of the overlapping with COPD. Early studies showed that only 3% of asthmatics developed their first symptoms of the disease after age 60. In the Cardiovascular Health Study, 4% of patients older than 65 years reported a current diagnosis of asthma. Another 4% had symptoms indicating "probable" asthma. More recently, one report stated that half of the asthmatic clinic patients over 65 had developed their asthma after age 40. The elderly asthmatic represented 20% of the population of that clinic. Clearly, new-onset asthma can occur at any age.

Our previous under-estimation of the prevalence of asthma may be partly caused by confusion with COPD because the two entities have a variety of clinical and functional similarities. A recent study identified 128 asthmatics with a mean age of 73 years (Bellia et al 2003). Only 53.1% had received the correct diagnosis of asthma, whereas 19.5% reported an incorrect diagnosis of COPD and/or emphysema; 27.3% had never had a diagnosis of their lung condition. Thus, 1 in 5 elderly asthmatic patients received the incorrect diagnosis of COPD, and 1 in 4 found to have asthma had never before had any diagnosis made.

Clinical Presentation

Asthma occurring in the elderly is separated into two groups based on the age of onset. *Early-onset asthma* has its initial presentation at any point before age 65. It is characterized by more severe, irreversible disease and a higher incidence of atopy. *Late-onset asthma* is defined as asthma in which the first symptoms appear after age 65. Patients with late-onset asthma may have better pulmonary function and airflow obstruction that is more easily reversible than in patients with early-onset disease. However, a subset of these elderly asthmatics has more resistant and less reversible disease. Characteristically, allergy history is negative in patients with late-onset asthma.

Older patients with asthma tend to report significantly greater symptom frequency than younger patients, but they are less likely to have nocturnal awakenings and asthma attacks. Daily cough and sputum production are more frequent in the aged. Also, there are more emergency room visits, unscheduled office visits, and increased hospitalizations compared with younger asthmatics. Many older-onset asthmatics report their first attack after an upper respiratory tract infection.

When the elderly patient presents with symptoms of cough, dyspnea, and wheezing, physicians often fail to consider the correct diagnosis, but instead attribute the symptoms to aging. Comorbid conditions such as chronic sinusitis, gastroesophageal reflux disease (GERD), and aspiration seen in this group can simulate and exacerbate asthma. In addition, an elderly asthmatic's perception of his or her disease is often poor: 60% of asthmatics have no correlation between their symptoms and objective measurements of lung function; 61% of patients who met current criteria of moderate asthma considered themselves totally or well controlled; and 32% with severe disease gave the same response (Boushey et al 2002).

Diagnosis

The diagnosis of asthma in the elderly is often difficult to establish. It is problematic, at times, to separate asthma from COPD, and they may coexist in the same individual. The boundary between the two diseases is often blurred; distinguishing between them is particularly difficult in older patients, especially those who have been smokers.

Laboratory testing is often unrevealing. The serum IgE level, which declines with age, is elevated in only 20% of asthmatic elderly, and skin testing is usually negative. Sputum and peripheral eosinophilia is often found, however, and may support the diagnosis of asthma.

Pulmonary function testing represents the most available and practical tool in obstructive airway diseases. This objective measurement of lung function is sadly underutilized by the medical community, and this is especially true in the elderly. This lack of testing contributes to the delay and absence of diagnosis in older patients. The testing of lung function is essential because of the decreased perception of dyspnea and the age-related decline in pulmonary function in the elderly. Yet in one study, less than one half of patients with the onset of asthma after age 65 had spirometry measurements after the diagnosis was suspected. Only two spirometric measurements have clinical relevance, the forced expiratory volume in 1 second (FEV_1) and the forced vital capacity (FVC) or its surrogate, FEV_6. The ratio between FEV_1/FVC is normally >0.7. When less, this suggests an obstructive disorder. When high, this often indicates a restrictive disorder (see Chapter 9).

Currently, the objective response to an inhaled bronchodilator is used to separate COPD (fixed airway obstruction) from asthma (reactive airways). The American Thoracic Society recommends that 12% improvement in either FEV_1 or FVC demonstrates reversibility, as long as the absolute magnitude of improvement in either measurement is at least 200 mL. However, using responsiveness to bronchodilators to separate COPD and asthma may result in an incorrect diagnosis. While the majority of asthmatics do show responsiveness, the early-onset elderly asthmatic may develop fixed airway obstruction and be classified as having COPD. Conversely, one study demonstrated a mean FEV_1 increase of 12.3% in response to an inhaled bronchodilator in a group of COPD patients (Bellia et al 2003). Spirometry studies will clearly establish the presence of airway abnormalities. Once airflow obstruction is established, it then becomes the clinician's role to identify the disease responsible for the obstructive process.

Treatment

In addition to the infrequency of correct diagnosis of asthma in the elderly, a more alarming problem is that even after a correct diagnosis, asthma is often undertreated. Studies have shown that the elderly asthmatic is given less aggressive therapy both on an outpatient basis and in the hospital, despite the fact that this group has more persistent and more severe disease which needs an aggressive, continued treatment program for control. Furthermore, the elderly are more likely to delay seeking medical attention and treatment once their asthma begins to worsen, which then compounds the problem.

Clinical practice guidelines for asthma treatment were first published in the United States in 1991. In 2002 the National Asthma Education and Prevention Program updated their 1997 recommendations. These guidelines, which have been widely circulated to clinicians, apply to both younger and older asthmatics (Table 11-2).

For persistent asthma (symptoms at least more than two times per week), the anti-inflammatory controller medication of choice is an inhaled

Table 11-2 Asthma Treatment by Severity of Disease

Mild intermittent asthma

Symptoms: ≤2×/wk; nighttime symptoms: ≤2×/mo; FEV_1 and PEFR ≥80% predicted; PEFR variability <20%.

Treatment: Inhaled short-acting β_2-agonist pm.

Mild persistent asthma

Symptoms: >2×/wk and <1×/d; nighttime symptoms: >2×/mo but ≤1×/wk; FEV_1 and PEFR ≥80% predicted; PEFR variability 20-30%.

Treatment: Begin anti-inflammatory therapy; inhaled corticosteroids are preferred or consider a leukotriene pathway modifier or cromolyn. Short-acting β_2-agonist pm for quick relief, but increased use means need for additional controller therapy.

Moderate persistent asthma

Symptoms: daily; nighttime symptoms: >1×/wk; FEV_1 and PEFR 60-80% predicted; PEFR variability >30%.

Treatment: Add long-acting β-agonist. If symptoms still persist, increase dose of inhaled corticosteroid, add leukotriene pathway modifier, or consider theophylline. Continue short-acting β_2-agonist for acute relief.

Severe persistent asthma

Symptoms: continual; limited physical activity; frequent exacerbations; frequent nighttime symptoms; FEV_1 or PEFR ≤60% predicted; PEFR variability >30%.

Treatment: Inhaled corticosteroids; long-acting β_2-agonist; theophylline; oral corticosteroids.

FEV_1 = forced expiratory volume in one second; PEFR = peak expiratory flow rate.

Adapted from National Asthma Education and Prevention Program, National Institutes of Health; 1997.

corticosteroid. No other medication is as effective as the corticosteroids in improving asthma outcomes. For moderate persistent and severe persistent asthma, the addition of a long-acting beta-agonist to the inhaled corticosteroid is recommended because strong evidence consistently indicates this drug combination improves asthma outcomes. The addition of a leukotriene modifier, theophylline, or doubling the dose of an inhaled steroid also improves outcomes, but not to the degree provided by the steroid/long-acting beta-agonist combination. Despite the above recommendation, a study found that only 30% of elderly asthmatics were receiving inhaled steroids (Enright et al 1999) .

With the use of low-to-moderate dosages of inhaled steroids, side effects are few. Oral moniliasis and vocal cord myopathy (leading to hoarseness) are the most common. Cataracts, glaucoma, hypothalamic-pituitary-adrenal axis suppression, and fractures have been reported with high-dose inhaled and oral corticosteroids but are usually not clinically significant with the lower doses in standard use.

The short-acting beta-agonists have long been the agents of choice for asthma rescue medicine. The elderly have a decrease in beta-receptor function. However, because of their past long-term track record, the short-acting beta-agonists are used in older patients. Tachycardia and tremor are associated with their use, either of which may present a problem for the patient. More recently, they have also been associated with an increased death rate resulting from ventricular arrhythmias in older patients with concomitant coronary artery disease. Because of this finding, their use in the elderly should be monitored. Earlier studies have found decreased asthma control and increased bronchial reactivity with regular usage, and the short-acting beta-agonists are currently recommended for as-needed rather than regular usage. The Rule of Twos has become an excellent guide to short-acting beta-agonist use: no more than 2 times per week rescue use; no more than 2 refills per year; and no more than 2 uses per month for nocturnal symptoms. A requirement for more frequent usage indicates the need to intensify the patient's maintenance regimen.

The elderly often have underlying diseases requiring treatments that have the potential to worsen their asthma. Every asthmatic should be warned about the use of aspirin and non-steroidal anti-inflammatory agents that can precipitate an attack in individuals with aspirin sensitivity and/or full-blown triad asthma (the combination of asthma, nasal polyps, and aspirin sensitivity).

Beta-blockers, which are commonly prescribed in this age group for CHF, hypertension, and angina, have long been known to increase airway resistance in COPD and exacerbate asthma. Even beta-blocking eye drops used for glaucoma can cause a significant problem. Cardioselective beta-blockers are less likely to cause bronchospasm than the non-cardioselective agents, but at higher doses may still precipitate bronchospasm. Physicians should closely monitor patients with airways disease when they are on beta-blocking agents.

Special attention should to be given to the elderly asthmatic when addressing a therapeutic program. These individuals may have problems not encountered in a younger asthmatic. Memory loss is common and may lead to poor adherence with the outlined program. Financial resources often limit patients' ability to obtain expensive medications. Physical problems with the hands can limit the use of delivery devices, and learning the inhaler technique is often a challenge. Elderly patients often live alone and have little support to help them with the above problems. The conscientious physician or another member of the health care team should provide specific written instructions, including dosing schedules and rescue instructions. Visiting nurses may assist in evaluating the home situation and making recommendations that will help the patient adhere to the therapeutic regimen. Additionally, elderly asthmatics may need to be seen more frequently than their younger counterparts to monitor their status, check on their inhaler technique, and carefully review their medication and the patient's adherence to the recommended regimen.

Clinical Outcomes and Prognosis

Remissions in asthma are seen commonly in the second decade of life, but are much less common in older age groups. One study of asthmatics over age 70 who were nonsmokers showed that none had a complete remission. The elderly asthmatic has more severe and persistent disease and is twice as likely to be hospitalized as a younger asthmatic. This group also has a higher death rate; 54% of the deaths from asthma between 1993 and 1995 were in patients 65 and older, and 75% of deaths from asthma in patients who were hospitalized occurred in patients over 55 years old (Diette et al 2002). These statistics should not discourage the physician. Rather, they should heighten suspicion of an asthma diagnosis and the need to institute aggressive care to control the disease.

Chronic Obstructive Pulmonary Disease

Definition

COPD is an all-inclusive and relatively nonspecific term that is applied to a spectrum of diseases that include chronic bronchitis, emphysema, and asthmatic bronchitis. The cardinal symptoms are chronic cough, mucus hypersecretion, dyspnea on exertion, and occasional wheeze. It is characterized by progressive airflow obstruction, which is demonstrated by a progressive reduction in expiratory airflow as judged by simple spirometry (forced expiratory volume in 1 second, FEV_1), and which is not completely reversible (Table 11-3). Lung hyperinflation occurs in the majority of patients.

Etiology

COPD results from inflammatory damage to the conducting airways, both large and small, and loss of elastic recoil due to damage of alveolar structures. The loss of elastic recoil and increased airways resistance due to inflammatory, fibrotic, and remodeling processes reduce expiratory airflow, which is a hallmark of disease severity and a predictor of prognosis. The most common cause of COPD is cigarette smoking.

Treatment

Current pharmacologic therapy consists of bronchodilators of the beta-adrenergic agonist, anticholinergic, and theophylline classes. Common drugs in use are albuterol, formoterol, salmeterol, ipratropium, and tiotropium by inhalation, and theophylline products taken orally. Anti-inflammatory therapy is often added with inhaled glucocorticoids. This therapy of COPD offers modest but significant symptomatic and physiologic benefits.

Only smoking cessation and supplemental oxygen administration have been proven to restrain or improve the natural history of COPD. Complete and permanent smoking cessation is the only intervention that improves FEV_1 in a sustained manner. Smoking cessation is most effective in early disease, but it is extremely difficult to implement and maintain in patients because of the addictive properties of nicotine.

Table 11-3 Spirometric Classification of COPD

Severity	Post-BD FEV_1/FVC	FEV_1, % of predicted
Mild	<70%	>80%
Moderate	<70%	50-80%
Severe	<70%	30-50%
Very severe	<70%	<30%

BD = bronchodilator.

Adapted from American Thoracic Society. Standards for the diagnosis and care of patients with COPD. Am J Resp Crit Care Med. 1995;152:S77-120.

Supplemental oxygen administration has utility in hypoxemic patients who have late-stage disease (see Chapter 13). Supplemental oxygen appears to work by forestalling the cardiovascular complications associated with cor pulmonale. Adjunctive therapies include exercise and respiratory vaccines. Nutritional supplements and antidepressants are often helpful. Lung volume reduction surgery offers benefit in selected patients with advanced COPD. Patient selection for lung volume reduction surgery or lung transplantation is best done in consultation with a pulmonologist.

COPD is associated with short, intermittent periods (1-3 weeks) of worsening symptoms that are termed *exacerbations*. Although an exacerbation is difficult to define, patients exhibit increased cough with increased sputum volume and purulence, shortness of breath, and loss of energy. Viral respiratory infection probably plays a larger role than bacterial infection in COPD exacerbations. Bacterial superinfection may lead to more severe exacerbations. Mild exacerbations are typically treated with a short course of an antibiotic aimed at common respiratory pathogens, while more severe exacerbations require therapy with antibiotics, intensive bronchodilator regimens, and systemic glucocorticoids. Hospitalization is often necessary. It appears that exacerbations can be associated with irreversible decrements in lung function. More effective treatment of the inflammatory and hypersecretory nature of acute exacerbations may help reduce progressive loss of lung function.

Bronchodilators

Tiotropium is a long-acting anticholinergic bronchodilator that is now approved in the United States for treatment of patients with COPD. It is inhaled once daily as a dry powder. Ipratropium was the first of this class of compounds to achieve widespread use as a bronchodilator for treatment of COPD. Tiotropium provides significant bronchodilator activity for up to 24 hours following administration. The drug inhibits acetylcholine-induced bronchoconstriction in a dose-dependent manner. Side effects are minimal and consist mostly of dry mucous membranes. Urinary retention and ocular side effects appear to be rare with tiotropium.

In clinical trials comparing tiotropium with ipratropium and placebo, tiotropium resulted in superior improvement in FEV_1, less dyspnea, and fewer exacerbations. Tiotropium has been shown to reduce hyperinflation and thus improve vital capacity and expiratory flow. In the categories of serious adverse events and events leading to study discontinuation, a lower incidence was reported with tiotropium than with control medications. Phase 4 studies are evaluating the added bronchodilator efficacy of a combination of tiotropium and a long-acting beta-2 adrenergic agonist and a possible survival benefit conferred by tiotropium.

Anti-Inflammatory Therapy

Inhaled glucocorticoids improve symptoms and may reduce the number and severity of exacerbations. It is as yet unknown whether these drugs interrupt the progressive decline in FEV_1 characteristic of COPD. Patients who benefit most seem to be those with prominent bronchitic symptoms and those who show some reversibility of airway obstruction after inhaled bronchodilators. Inhaled corticosteroids may achieve their beneficial effect by suppressing mast cells and CD8+ lymphocytes. In the United States, the combination of fluticasone and salmeterol is approved for treatment of COPD.

In phosphodiesterase-4 inhibitors, the intracellular enzyme, phosphodiesterase-4 (PDE-4), has a pro-inflammatory effect by metabolizing cyclic AMP. PDE-4 inhibitors relax smooth muscle cells, suppress inflammatory cell activation, and modulate the activity of pulmonary nerves. Several drugs of this class have entered phase III study. These drugs are oral agents dosed once or twice daily. Gastrointestinal side effects are the most common problems associated with this class of drugs. These drugs remain under study.

A number of leukotriene inhibitors have been synthesized and several are approved for treatment of asthma. As yet, none of these agents has been approved for treatment of COPD, although they are sometimes prescribed for this purpose.

Future Trends in Therapy

The ultimate goal of COPD therapy is to develop a drug that interrupts lung destruction, effects lung repair, and restores alveolar integrity. Retinoids are chemical derivatives of vitamin A. The finding that retinoic acid lessened emphysema in rats given intratracheal elastase raised great hope for retinoids as therapeutic agents in humans with COPD. Retinoids have been shown to modulate elastin gene expression in cultured fibroblasts and also to influence alveolar formation in rats in vivo. Human trials have not shown a clinical benefit from retinoids. Liver toxicity is also a problem.

Mucus hypersecretion and the inability to clear secretions from the airways are prominent manifestations of COPD. Drugs that reduce mucus hypersecretion or aid in clearance of mucus could lead to substantial symptomatic improvement in patients with COPD. Several mucoactive drugs are under current investigation.

Summary

Asthma in the elderly is far more common than previously suspected and is frequently overlooked or misdiagnosed. It may reflect early-onset asthma that has progressed, or it may present as new-onset disease. Clinicians must become more proactive in their evaluation of the elderly. Pulmonary function testing should be considered an essential part of the diagnostic evaluation of patients with respiratory symptoms. Once asthma is diagnosed, patients need special and personalized care because of their more persistent and severe disease and their diminished ability to cope with their situation physically, financially, and emotionally.

Therapeutic possibilities are expanding for COPD, but many of these new drugs are still being evaluated and remain unproven therapies. Tiotropium and an inhaled glucocorticoid in the combination product fluticasone and salmeterol are already approved and offer symptomatic relief and some long-term value in moderate or advanced stages of disease. Studies are in progress to determine if these two classes of drug will interrupt the progressive decline in FEV_1. New drugs, including novel anti-inflammatory drugs, mucus secretion inhibitors, and especially drugs that stimulate lung growth and repair such as retinoids, may offer even greater therapeutic utility. Some of these new drugs may directly inhibit lung destruction or enhance lung repair and regeneration.

BIBLIOGRAPHY AND SUGGESTED READING

I. ASTHMA

Bellia V, Battaglia S, Catalano F, et al. Aging and disability affect misdiagnosis of COPD in elderly asthmatics. Chest. 2003;123:1066-72. *Evaluation of misdiagnosis of COPD in elderly asthmatics.*

Boushey HA, Stempel DA. Foreword. Asthma in America. J Allergy Clin Immunol. 2002;115:s479-s481.

Braman SS. Asthma in the elderly. Clin Geriatr Med. 2003;19:57-75. *Comprehensive review of the presentation and treatment of asthma in the elderly.*

Diette GB, Krishnan JA, Dominici F, et al. Asthma in older patients: factors associated with hospitalization. Arch Int Med. 2002;162:1123-37. *Review of factors associated with hospitalization.*

Enright PL, McClelland RL, Newman AB, et al. Underdiagnosis and undertreatment of asthma in the elderly. Chest. 1999;116:603-13. *Presentation of data from elderly asthmatic patients enrolled in the Cardiovascular Health Study.*

Global Initiative for Asthma. Global Strategy for Asthma Management and Prevention. National Institute of Health, National Heart, Lung & Blood Institute. Publication 95-3654, 1995;1-71. *Goals and objectives of the National Asthma Education and Prevention Program (NAEPP).*

National Asthma Education and Prevention Program (NAEPP). Expert Panel Report: Guidelines for the Diagnosis and Management of Asthma – Update on Selected Topics 2002. Bethesda, MD: National Institutes of Health. July 2002. NIH publication 02-5075. *Update of the NAEPP.*

Quadrelli SA, Roncoroni A. Features of asthma in the elderly. J Asthma. 2001;38:377-89. *Review discussing the incidence, severity, treatment, and problems encountered in the elderly asthmatic.*

II. CHRONIC OBSTRUCTIVE PULMONARY DISEASE

Casaburi R, Mahler DA, Jones PW, et al. A long-term evaluation of once-daily inhaled tiotropium in chronic obstructive pulmonary disease. Eur Respir J. 2002;19:217-24. *Patients receiving tiotropium had improved symptom relief and fewer exacerbations.*

Hanania NA, Darken P, Horstman D, et al. The efficacy and safety of fluticasone propionate (250 µg)/salmeterol (50 µg) combined in the Diskus inhaler for the treatment of COPD. Chest. 2003;124:834-43. *Combined fluticasone and salmeterol was superior to either drug alone in improving FEV_1 and peak exploratory flow over a 6-month study.*

Pauwels R. Inhaled glucocorticoids and COPD: how full is the glass?. Am J Resp Crit Care Med. 2002;165:1579-80. *Inhaled glucocorticoids give symptomatic relief and help prevent exacerbations.*

Pauwels RA, Buist AS, Calverley PM, et al. Global strategy for the diagnosis, management and prevention of chronic obstructive pulmonary disease. NHLBI/WHO Global Initiative for Chronic Obstructive Lung Disease (GOLD) Workshop Summary. Am J Respir Crit Care Med. 2001;163:1256-76.

Soriano JB, Vestbo J, Pride NB, et al. Survival in COPD patients after regular use of fluticasone propionate and salmeterol in general practice. Eur Respir J. 2002;20:819-25. *Retrospective report based on available evidence that the combined use of fluticasone with salmeterol had a survival benefit in moderate-to-advanced COPD.*

Vincken W, van Noord JA, Greefhorst AP, et al, on behalf of the Dutch/Belgian Tiotropium Study Group. Improved health outcomes in patients with COPD during one-year treatment with tiotropium. Eur Respir J. 2002; 9:209-16. *Patients treated with tiotropium had greater bronchodilation and symptom relief than patients receiving ipratropium or placebo.*

12 Intrathoracic Malignancies

L
ung cancer is the most common fatal malignancy in both men and
women. It occurs most often in the elderly; its incidence increases with
age, and the median age of presentation in the United States is about 67
years. Older age, however, should not be seen as a barrier to cancer treatment, nor should it be assumed that treatment will be less effective in older
than in younger patients. Surgical resection has approximately the same outcome in persons over the age of 70 as in younger individuals. Intrathoracic
malignancies considered in this chapter include primary lung cancer,
mesothelioma, secondary (metastatic) lung cancer, and sarcomas.

Primary Lung Cancer

Carcinoma of the lung is subdivided into non–small cell lung cancer
(NSCLC), representing about 75% of all primary carcinomas of the lung, and
small cell lung cancer (SCLC). NSCLC is further divided into squamous cell
carcinoma, adenocarcinoma (including bronchioloalveolar cell carcinoma),
and large cell carcinoma. Combinations may occur. Eighty-five percent of
cases of lung cancer are attributable to smoking, from either direct or passive
smoking. The cause of the other 15% is multifactorial, including genetic factors, occupational and environmental hazards, and other unknown hazards.
Unfortunately, no scientific or governmental society currently recommends
the early identification of lung cancer in the United States. By contrast,
screening for early lung carcinoma is the standard of care for all smokers over
the age of 45 in Japan. This has led to a major stage shift in diagnosis, early

recognition, and treatment in Japan, and a far better survival rate in screened than in non-screened patients.

Recent studies have shown that asymptomatic lung cancer can be identified in a very high-risk population of patients who consult their primary care physicians for any reason (Bechtel et al 2005). The cost of finding a new cancer was less than $12,000 (seven of the patients with airflow obstruction were found to have lung cancer in various stages). One half of the cancers were in early stages of the disease (i.e., 1A).

Diagnosis

Most patients who are diagnosed with lung cancer present with symptoms of advanced stages of disease. This accounts for approximately 75% of all cancers because of the way lung cancer is identified in the United States. Despite the importance of early diagnosis, lung cancer is often asymptomatic for one to several years before it becomes manifest on standard chest x-rays or CT scanning or by symptoms. But by this time the cancer has gone through many mutational changes, resulting in a progressively aggressive malignancy.

Common presentations are cough, often attributed to smoking; hemoptysis, which itself can be due to chronic bronchitis; and dyspnea, due to the underlying cancer, associated COPD, or pleural effusion. Extrapulmonary manifestations include CNS manifestations, supraclavicular node enlargement, bone pain, superior vena cava syndrome, and paraneoplastic syndromes.

Roentgenographic appearances include the solitary nodule, small peripheral nodules, hilar masses, and large parenchymal masses. Comments about each are appropriate.

- *Solitary nodules* (calcified or not calcified) even in endemic areas of fungal infections are most commonly benign. Even though lung cancer can present as a solitary pulmonary nodule (Figure 12-1), most pulmonary nodules are benign rather than malignant. The risk of malignancy increases with smoking history, age, and size of the nodule. Benign lesions of approximately 1 cm and smooth border are commonly seen on chest x-rays. An irregular border suggests malignancy, but the specificity and sensitivity of this observation are low. Small lesions are often missed. CT scanning is effective in identifying small cancers that are not visible on standard chest x-rays. CT and PET scanning may both be useful in differentiating malignant from benign disease, but the sensitivity and specificity of both scans are not high enough for diagnostic certainty. Although calcification

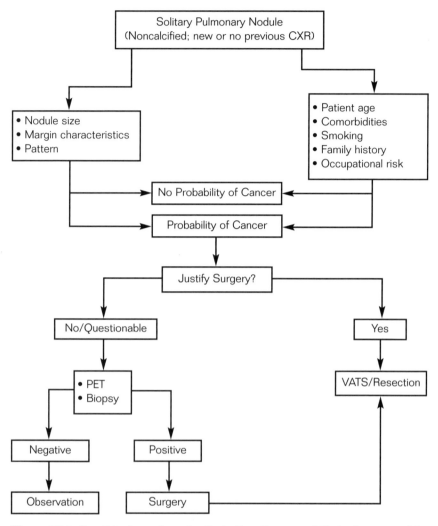

Figure 12-1 Algorithim for work-up of patient with solitary noncalcified pulmonary nodule.

within a nodule often suggests that the lesion is benign, this is true only for certain patterns of calcification. Other patterns of calcification, particularly eccentric calcification within a nodule, may be suggestive of malignancy. Work-up of the solitary nodule often begins with the general internist.

- *Small peripheral nodules* that are identified by CT are likely malignant if growth occurs within 6-12 months. These nodules are subject to further investigations, including needle aspiration or excisional biopsies such as video-assisted thoracic surgery

(VATS). Cavitary masses may represent slowly growing squamous cell carcinoma.

- *Hilar masses* are most commonly squamous cell carcinoma or small cell carcinoma and can be evaluated by CT, bronchoscopy, and biopsy.
- *Diffuse bilateral lymphangitic metastasis,* including the presence of Kerley B lines, is an advanced complication of both primary and metastatic lung cancer.

The use of PET and CT scanning for staging has increased our ability to judge who is resectable for potential cure. The PET scan is based on increased glucose metabolism, which is common in lung cancer but can occur in active granulomas or other active inflammatory processes. False-negative PET scans may occur in small bronchioloalveolar cancers and bronchial carcinoid tumors.

Unfortunately, the outcome for lung cancer will not change significantly until we adopt an approach of early identification and intervention, particularly in high-risk patients. This has become the standard of care in Japan. For this reason lung cancer survival in Japan at 5-10 years is comparable to that for other cancers such as breast, colon, and ovarian.

Lung cancer is five to six times more common in smokers with airflow obstruction (FEV_1 <80% of predicted) than in smokers with normal airflow. Thus, lung cancer should be suspected in patients with a strong family history of cancer, a history of smoking, a history of occupational or non-occupational exposure to other risk factors for lung cancer (e.g., radon, asbestos), and in those with airflow obstruction as identified by spirometry.

Standard diagnostic techniques for lung cancer include chest x-ray, thoracic CT, and fiberoptic bronchoscopy. Lung cancer is identified by chest x-ray and CT scanning, and confirmed by biopsy or surgical resection. While the chest x-ray can identify nodules greater than 1 cm in diameter, smaller lesions and those hidden by bony, mediastinal, and cardiac structures are often missed. Sputum cytology is helpful in identifying early central lesions, which are not seen on CT. Once a lesion is identified, previous CT and x-ray studies should be reviewed, and appropriate consultation obtained. If the lesion is of unknown duration, a 3-month period of observation may be followed and the appropriate study repeated at that time. If the lesion is new or has other characteristics suggestive of malignancy and observation seems inappropriate, a biopsy to confirm a tissue diagnosis should be done.

When establishing a tissue diagnosis, the approach that is least invasive and has the highest yield should be employed. At times, a direct surgical approach is best to provide better staging and to eliminate sampling error.

For newly diagnosed lung nodules and masses, bronchoscopy, transthoracic needle biopsy, or video-assisted thoracic surgery (VATS) is commonly used.

With smaller peripheral lesions (<2 cm) transthoracic biopsy or VATS is the procedure of choice. When patients present with atelectasis or if pulmonary infiltrates suspicious for endobronchial obstruction are suspected, fiberoptic bronchoscopy is indicated.

Two newer techniques for diagnosis merit separate discussion. First is the use of low-radiation-dose CT to screen patients at high risk for lung cancer. The technique is much more sensitive in identifying non-calcified pulmonary nodules than standard chest x-ray. Because of the rapid imaging capabilities (10-20 seconds for an entire study), costs can be low in rapid throughput centers. Second is the use of a special bronchoscope to detect dysplasia and carcinoma *in situ* by tissue autofluorescence. The Lung Imaging Fluorescence Endoscope (LIFE) takes advantage of the difference in autofluorescence between normal and dysplastic tissue when blue light (instead of white light) is utilized. The abnormal areas are then biopsied under direct vision and sent for histopathologic evaluation. Currently, this technology is only used in high-risk patients who have airflow obstruction, a heavy smoking history, and sputum atypia.

Staging

When lung cancer is diagnosed by sputum cytology, biopsy, or resection, staging is the next step. For non-small-cell carcinoma, staging is necessary to plan treatment and for prognostic purposes. A revised staging system offered by Mountain (1997) is presented in Table 12-1; the descriptors used in the staging system are presented in Table 12-2. CT scanning, positron emission tomography (PET) scans, and surgical exploration (mediastinoscopy or thoracotomy) are also used in staging. Surgery is appropriate for stages I to IIIA, depending on patient comorbidities. In general, prognosis worsens with advancing stages, as with all cancers.

A different staging system is used for small cell lung cancer. The disease is categorized as either "limited" (confined to one hemithorax) or "extensive" (disease is present outside the ipsilateral hemithorax). Because small cell carcinoma of the lung is generally considered to have at least microscopic dissemination by the time of detection, systemic chemotherapy is the mainstay of therapy for virtually all cases. For limited disease, however, radiotherapy is often added as part of a combined modality regimen. Radiotherapy is not an option for extensive disease.

Because of the high incidence of unsuspected advanced (stage III and IV) disease when lung cancer is initially diagnosed, a technique that could

Table 12-1 Staging of Lung Cancer

Number	TNM
0	Carcinoma in situ
IA	T1N0M0
IB	T2N0M0
IIA	T1N1M0
IIB	T2N1M0
	T3N0M0
IIIA	T3N1M0
	T1N2M0
	T2N2M0
	T3N2M0
IIIB	T4N0M0
	T4N1M0
	T4N2M0
	Any TN3M0
IV	Any T
	Any NM1

See Table 12-2 for TNM descriptors.
Staging is not relevant for occult carcinoma, designated TXN0M0. The uncommon superficial tumor of any size with its invasive component limited to the bronchial wall, which may extend proximal to the main bronchus, is also classified T1. Most pleural effusions associated with lung cancer are due to tumor. However, there are a few patients in whom multiple cytopathologic examinations of pleural fluid show no tumor. In these cases, the fluid is non-bloody and is not an exudate. When these elements and clinical judgment dictate that the effusion is not related to the tumor, the effusion should be excluded as a staging element and the patient's disease should be staged T1, T2 or T3. Pericardial effusion is classified according to the same rules. Separate metastatic tumor nodule(s) in the ipsilateral nonprimary-tumor lobe(s) of the lung also are classified M1.
From Mountain CF. Revisions in the International System for Staging Lung Cancer. Chest 1997;111:1710-7; with permission.

identify metastatic disease would be extremely helpful. CT scans may show enlarged nodes, but many times pathological correlation is not good. The PET technique is more accurate than CT for the staging of lung cancer. Fluorodeoxyglucose (FDG) is administered to the patient and has increased accumulation in malignant cells. The FDG PET scan identifies malignant nodes and metastatic disease that is unsuspected by conventional imaging. Solitary pulmonary nodules that have increased uptake of FDG are more likely to be malignant and require tissue diagnosis, while those that do not enhance may be observed for 3 months and then re-imaged with a chest x-ray or low-radiation-dose CT.

Mesothelioma

Mesotheliomas are rare and, when found in the elderly, occur in patients with asbestos-related occupational activities that took place in younger years. A pleural-based mass (or masses), usually with a pleural effusion, is the most

Table 12-2 TNM Descriptors

Primary tumor (T)	TX: Primary tumor cannot be assessed, or tumor proven by the presence of malignant cells in sputum or bronchial washings but not visualized by imaging or bronchoscopy
	TO: No evidence of primary tumor
	Tis: Carcinoma in situ
	T1: Tumor ≤3 cm in greatest dimension, surrounded by lung or visceral pleura, without bronchoscopic evidence of invasion more proximal than the lobar bronchus (i.e., not the main bronchus)
	T2: Tumor with any of the following features in size or extent: >3 cm in greatest dimension; involves main bronchus, >2 cm distal to the carina; invades the visceral pleura; associated with atelectasis or obstructive pneumonitis that extends to the hilar region but does not involve the entire lung
	T3: Tumor of any size that directly invades any of the following: chest wall (including superior sulcus tumors), diaphragm, mediastinal pleura, parietal pericardium; or tumor in the main bronchus <2 cm distal to the carina, but without involvement of the carina; or associated atelectasis or obstructive pneumonitis of the entire lung
	T4: Tumor of any size that invades any of the following: mediastinum, heart, great vessels, trachea, esophagus, vertebral body, carina; or tumor with a malignant pleural or pericardial effusion, or with satellite tumor nodule(s) within the ipsilateral primary-tumor lobe of the lung
Regional lymph nodes (N)	NX: Regional lymph nodes cannot be assessed
	N0: No regional lymph node metastasis
	N1: Metastasis to ipsilateral peribronchial and/or ipsilateral hilar lymph nodes, and intrapulmonary nodes involved by direct extension of the primary tumor
	N2: Metastasis to ipsilateral mediastinal and/or subcarinal lymph node(s)
	N3: Metastasis to contralateral mediastinal, contralateral hilar, ipsilateral or contralateral scalene, or supraclavicular lymph node(s)
Distant metastasis (M)	MX: Presence of distant metastasis cannot be assessed
	M0: No distant metastasis
	M1: Distant metastasis present

From Mountain CF. Revisions in the International System for Staging Lung Cancer. Chest. 1997;111:1710-7; with permission.

common presentation, which explains the typical symptoms of dyspnea and, often, chest pain at presentation.

Secondary Lung Cancer

The secondary spread of cancer to the lung can be from a variety of primary tumors, including the lung itself. Metastases may occur either by direct extension or by lymphatic or blood stream spread. Multiple round nodules or pleural effusions are the most common roentgenographic manifestations. The lung's capillaries are an efficient filtering system, and nearly the entire cardiac output traverses the pulmonary capillaries. Thus it is natural that metastatic spread from many sites is common. The most frequent primary sites are breast, colon, ovarian, renal, other gastrointestinal organs, thyroid, and testicle.

Sarcomas

Sarcomas, often originating in bone and joint, commonly metastasize to the lungs. Their presence suggests an ominous prognosis. Primary lymphomas of the lung and pulmonary manifestations of generalized lymphomas are fairly common in high-risk groups such as patients with AIDS and patients with extensive radiation exposure from either treatment or environmental causes such as radiation disasters.

Treatment

A complete discussion of the treatment of lung cancer is beyond the scope of this chapter. Decisions about specific patients are often best made by a multidisciplinary team that includes a pulmonologist, a thoracic surgeon, an oncologist, and a radiation therapist. Treatment of NSCLC depends upon the staging of the disease and the functional status of the patient, rather than the patient's chronologic age. Surgery is preferred for localized disease in the patient whose functional status suggests that (s)he can tolerate lung resectional surgery. Other treatment modalities involve radiation therapy, chemotherapy, combined modality therapy, and photodynamic therapy. Survival is being improved with new chemotherapies. Oral therapies are just emerging, but chemotherapy remains in the province of the oncologist or experienced pulmonologist who treats advanced lung cancer.

A recent editorial by an expert pulmonologist/oncologist emphasizes the increased effectiveness and improved survival and quality of life for established and newer chemotherapy. Response rates have improved to above

50% with 20-30% of patients with metastatic NSCLC surviving >2 years (Ruckdeschel 2006). Treatment of small cell carcinoma is by chemotherapy, radiation therapy, or a combination of the two. Surgery is rarely curative. Improved chemotherapy for mesothelioma is emerging.

BIBLIOGRAPHY AND SUGGESTED READING

Bechtel JJ, Kelley WA, Coons TA, et al. Lung cancer detection in patients with airflow obstruction identified in a primary care outpatient practice. Chest. 2005;127:1140-5. *Report of a community identification project for unsuspected lung cancer in high-risk patients, identified by a simple questionnaire.*

Bechtel JJ, Kelley WR, Petty TL, et al. Outcome of 51 patients with roentgenographically occult lung cancer detected by sputum cytologic testing: a community hospital program. Arch Intern Med. 1994;154:975-80. *Discusses the outcome of patients diagnosed solely on the basis of sputum cytology.*

Bechtel JJ, Petty TL, Saccomanno G. Five-year survival and later outcome of patients with x-ray occult lung cancer detected by sputum cytology. Lung Cancer. 2000;30:1-7. *Follow-up of the above article showing a greater than 50% survival in lung cancer diagnosed by sputum cytology.*

Henschke CI. Early lung cancer action project: overall design and findings from baseline screening. Cancer. 2000;89:2474-82. *Elaboration on the original early lung cancer identification project using CT reported in Lancet (1999;354:94-105).*

Henschke CI, Naidich DP, Yankelevitz DF, et al. Early lung cancer action project: initial findings on repeat screenings. Cancer. 2001;92:153-9. *Follow-up on the original screening study in Lancet (see above).*

Mountain CF. Revisions in the International System for Staging Lung Cancer. Chest. 1997;111:1710-7.

Ost D, Fein A. Evaluation and management of the solitary pulmonary nodule. Am J Respir Crit Care Med. 2000;162:782-7. *Brief commentary on the state of the art in the diagnosis and management of the solitary nodule. PET scanning has increased in use since this publication.*

Petty TL. The early diagnosis of lung cancer. Dis Mon. 2001;47:204-64. *Comprehensive review of the importance of early diagnosis and the technologies involved.*

Ruckdeschel JC. Second-line chemotherapy for non-small-cell lung cancer. Chest. 2006;129:840-2.

13 Home Treatment of Chronic Respiratory Disorders

ome treatment of chronic pulmonary disorders, particularly with oxygen, has improved dramatically in the past 30 years. This has enhanced the length and quality of life of all patients, including the elderly. The major technical components of home care are long-term oxygen therapy (LTOT) and mechanical ventilation.

Long-Term Oxygen Therapy

LTOT has been shown to improve quality of life, increase longevity, and reduce hospitalizations in hypoxemic patients with chronic obstructive pulmonary disease (COPD). More than 1.3 million patients in the United States are receiving LTOT. In the 1960s, Petty and others in the Denver group treated ambulatory hypoxic patients using portable liquid oxygen systems and documented reversal of pulmonary hypertension and erythrocytosis. The ability to ambulate while breathing oxygen was shown to improve physical conditioning and psychological issues compared with home-bound patients who were tethered to bulky oxygen tanks. This section focuses on the practical aspects of LTOT, including indications, the oxygen prescription, and oxygen delivery systems.

Indications and Requirements

The most common indication for LTOT is for treatment of advanced COPD associated with hypoxemia, but patients with a variety of respiratory disorders may also benefit. These may include patients with chronic interstitial lung disease, neuromuscular diseases, chest wall deformities, and patients with congestive heart failure. The Center for Medicare and Medicaid Services (CMS, formerly the Healthcare Financing Administration, HCFA) classifies oxygen therapy as "durable medical equipment," and regulates reimbursements for home ambulatory oxygen in Medicare and Medicaid patients. Most third-party payers follow the CMS indications and requirements for LTOT. Table 13-1 outlines the indications and requirements for LTOT reimbursement by CMS.

Baseline measurement of arterial blood gases (ABG) is the usual means of assessing the need for oxygen therapy. Pulse oximetry is an efficient and a noninvasive method to estimate arterial oxygenation and can be used while patients are exercising or during sleep. Oximetry should be used as an adjunct to ABGs in evaluating the need for LTOT. Pulse oximetry has limitations and may under- or over-estimate oxygenation in some patients (Table 13-2).

The Oxygen Prescription

The oxygen prescription (Figure 13-1) should specify the following:

- Liter flow rate while at rest, walking, exercising, and during sleep
- Continuous or intermittent oxygen (for example, during exercise or sleep)
- Hours used per day
- *Oxygen delivery equipment*: stationary, portable, or both
- *Delivery systems*: nasal cannula, mask, conserving device, transtracheal oxygen

There is a consensus that oxygen flow rates should be sufficient to maintain arterial oxygen saturation by pulse oximetry (SpO_2) of 90-92% at all times and that oxygen should be used for at least 15 hours per day.

Worsening hypoxemia may require an increased rate of oxygen delivery during exacerbations of COPD, during air flight, and with changes in altitude. Significant nocturnal hypoxemia occurs in 25-45% of patients with severe COPD. Overnight SpO_2 monitoring may be used to titrate oxygen dosing during sleep but may not be practical in all cases. The general consensus is that the hypoxemic COPD patient should increase the liter flow rate by 1 L/min during sleep if oximetry cannot be performed. Nocturnal oxygen therapy is indicated in patients with right-sided heart failure, cor pulmonale, or erythrocytosis (hematocrit equal to or greater than 55%).

**Table 13-1 Medicare Indications and Requirements
for Long-Term Home Oxygen Therapy**

Indications

- $PaO_2 \leq 55$ mm Hg while breathing ambient air

- $SaO_2 \leq 88\%$ while breathing ambient air

- PaO_2 between 56 and 59 mm Hg or $SaO_2 \geq 89\%$ with any of the following:

  - Cor pulmonale by EKG
  - Right heart failure
  - Erythrocytosis (hematocrit above 55%)

- $PaO_2 \geq 60$ mm Hg or $SaO_2 \geq 90\%$, if there is compelling medical justification (such as comfort therapy for terminal cancer)

Requirements

- Optimal medical management required before certification

- Measurement of arterial blood gases or oxygen saturation by a qualified laboratory

- Measurements of PaO_2 and SaO_2 made no more than 2 days before hospital discharge

- Completion of Certification of Medical Necessity (CMN) (Form HCFA-484) by physician or staff

- If the PaO_2 is between 56 and 59 mm Hg or SaO_2 is $\geq 89\%$, the testing of arterial blood gases or oxygen saturation must be repeated in 60-120 days.

- Patients receiving LTOT must be recertified in 12 months.

- Patients receiving portable oxygen must be mobile in the home and regularly go 50 feet or more from the delivery system.

Table 13-2 Limitations of Pulse Oximetry

- May falsely underestimate hypoxemia

- Does not measure ventilation

- Inaccurate in patients with hemoglobinopathies:

  - Carboxyhemoglobin: falsely high SpO_2
  - Methemoglobin: falsely high SpO_2
  - Sickle hemoglobin: falsely high or falsely low

- Hypoperfusion/vasospasm: falsely low values

Oxygen Therapy During Exercise

Hypoxemic patients invariably decrease their physical activity as the underlying disease process progresses, leading to decreasing mobility and deconditioning. This may start a downhill spiral, both from a physical and a psychological perspective. Studies have shown that supplemental oxygen during exercise allows for increased activity, improved conditioning, and

---

Name _____   **Date** _____

Address   _____

                     _____

Diagnosis   _____

Resting PaO$_2$ _____mm Hg   SaO$_2$ _____%

Exercise PaO$_2$ _____mm Hg   SaO$_2$ _____%

Oxygen Flow Rate

Resting   _____L/ min   Minimum hours/day _____

During Sleep   _____L/min

Walking   _____L/min

Delivery System

                 Nasal Cannula___   Conserving Device___   Mask___

                 CPAP___   BiLevel___   Transtracheal___

Oxygen Source

                 Stationary___   Stationary and Portable___

                 Stationary and Ambulatory___

                 Ambulatory only___   Portable only___

                 (signed) _____ M.D./ D.O.

Figure 13-1 Sample home oxygen prescription.

improved quality of life. Also, supplemental oxygen during exercise can prevent or reduce increases in pulmonary artery pressure and pulmonary vascular resistance.

Titration during the "6-minute walk" can determine oxygen requirements during exercise. The goal of therapy is to maintain a SpO$_2$ equal to or greater than 90% at rest or while walking.

Continuous-Flow Delivery Systems

LTOT is generally supplied by three types of continuous-flow delivery systems:

- Oxygen concentrators
- Liquid oxygen devices and reservoirs
- Compressed gas cylinders

Oxygen Concentrators

Oxygen concentrators are electrically powered devices using molecular sieves to filter and concentrate oxygen molecules from ambient air. These devices generate concentrations of oxygen varying from 90% to 93% with maximal flow rates of 3-5 L/min. The fraction of inspired oxygen (FIO_2) decreases as flow rate increases. Concentrators are the most cost-efficient of the stationary oxygen delivery systems, but they are dependent on electrical power. Oxygen cylinders are required for back-up in the event of electrical power failure.

Oxygen concentrators were formerly large-console appliances that remained stationary, typically in the bedroom, with hoses up to 50 ft long supplying oxygen to nasal cannulas. Today, there are five battery-powered concentrators small enough for practical use while traveling in automobiles, on boats, and on aircraft. These portable systems are compact and weigh 5 to 17 lb. The 17-lb device (Eclipse) gives a continuous oxygen flow up to 3 L/min. All use batteries with an approximately 2-hour life plus extended power sources. Oxygen-conserving devices make oxygen delivery more efficient.

Effective September 5, 2006, portable oxygen concentrators approved by the Federal Aviation Administration may be carried and used on board aircraft. Non-approved concentrators that meet carry-on size and weight requirements may be brought on board with the batteries removed, or they may be transported as checked baggage. Patients travelling by air should check with their airline for information on current regulations.

Liquid Oxygen Systems

Liquid oxygen reservoirs provide a home source of oxygen at 2 L/min for 3-4 weeks. They may be used to refill portable liquid oxygen systems, which have become the most widely used means of portable administration of oxygen.

Oxygen systems that allow the patient to be fully active—to leave the home to work and to participate in recreational activities—are critical in the physical and mental rehabilitation of hypoxemic patients. Requirements for portable oxygen systems are as follows:

- The device must have the size and weight to allow the patient to carry it.
- It must provide oxygen delivery to the patient for a reasonable time period.
- It must be cost-effective.

Portable liquid oxygen systems are the most practical ambulatory delivery systems. Portable liquid oxygen tanks weigh 6-10 lb and can deliver 2 L/min of nasal oxygen for up to 10 hours before being refilled from a stationary liquid oxygen reservoir. The HELiOS and Spirit systems further reduce the weight and increase the portability of the device by combining the storage capacity of a liquid system with a pulsed oxygen-conserving device (see below). Portable devices weigh as little as 3.6 lb and provide a flow rate of 2 L/min for up to 8-10 hours.

Compressed Gas Cylinders

Compressed gas cylinders do not require an electrical source but are impractical for continuous or intermittent home use. An H-size cylinder weighs approximately 150 lb and can provide up to 57 hours of oxygen at a flow rate of 2 L/min.

Small, "lightweight," refillable oxygen cylinders are readily available and inexpensive but are relatively heavy, weighing 13-17 lb, and generally require a cart to contain the small E-sized cylinder. This system is cumbersome and lasts only approximately 5½ hours at 2 L/min. Pressurizing units have recently been developed to fill small oxygen cylinders from home-based oxygen concentrators.

Oxygen-Conserving Delivery Systems

The continuous-flow nasal cannula is the standard device used for administrating oxygen. It is well-tolerated by the patient with minimal side effects, but it is inefficient. In an effort to increase the range and reduce the weight of ambulatory oxygen systems, conserving devices were developed. Three classes of conservers are available:

- Reservoir cannulas
- Demand pulsing devices
- Transtracheal devices

Reservoir Cannulas

Reservoir cannula oxygen conservers function by storing oxygen during exhalation. With the next inhalation the stored oxygen plus oxygen from the delivery source is delivered to the alveoli, increasing oxygen saturation while reducing flow rates and thus conserving oxygen. These cannulas are available in two configurations: the Oximizer and the Pendent.

The Oximizer uses a "nasal pillow" cannula with a reservoir beneath the nose storing oxygen during exhalation along with the continuous flow from the liquid oxygen source. The Pendent cannula stores oxygen during exhalation in a reservoir residing on the anterior chest. The Oximizer tends to be more comfortable for most patients but is also more conspicuous and therefore less cosmetically desirable. Conversely, the Pendent is less noticeable but may be less comfortable for some patients.

Demand Pulsing Devices

Demand pulsing conservers deliver a pulse of oxygen only during inhalation. As the patient inhales, a solenoid in the system rapidly opens and closes, delivering a bolus of pure oxygen to the airways during the earliest phase of inhalation. These devices are used most commonly with liquid systems (e.g., HELiOS, Spirit). They are also intrinsic to portable oxygen concentrators. They may be used with compressed gas cylinders as well.

Transtracheal Devices

Transtracheal oxygen (TTO) delivery is an alternative to nasal cannulas, one with its own advantages and disadvantages. It involves the insertion of a tracheal catheter percutaneously and is used in a minority of patients on LTOT.

The advantages of TTO are:

- Improves compliance.
- Decreases oxygen use by 37-58% compared with continuous nasal oxygen.
- Allows adequate PaO_2 that may not be achievable in some patients by nasal cannula.
- Avoids irritation secondary to the nasal cannula.
- Improves exercise endurance and decreases dyspnea.
- Is less conspicuous and more acceptable cosmetically than a nasal cannula.

There are disadvantages also. Transtracheal oxygen delivery:

- Requires an invasive procedure, special training by the physician placing the catheter, staff monitoring, and follow-up with the patient.
- Has potential for infection, especially in immunocompromised patients.
- Is contraindicated in patients on warfarin or with coagulopathies.
- Is contraindicated in patients with vocal cord paralysis, severe obesity, frequent COPD exacerbations, and those requiring high-dose corticosteroids (>30 mg prednisone per day).

- Has patency that may be compromised by mucus balls.
- Requires commitment by patient and caregiver to maintain the transtracheal catheter.

Humidification

Humidification during oxygen administration with a nasal cannula is unnecessary when the flow is ≤5 L/min, unless the patient is receiving oxygen by tracheostomy or transtracheal catheter. Studies have shown no difference in adverse effects when bubble humidifiers are compared with no humidification. An exception may be made in certain situations with extremely low ambient humidity, or in patients with copious secretions.

Oxygen During Air Travel

Air travel is considered safe for most hypoxemic patients with stable chronic respiratory disease, provided they increase flow rates by 1-2 L/min during flights. Patients with PaO_2 levels of 70 mm Hg or greater should be able to travel safely without supplemental oxygen.

The FAA has approved five portable oxygen concentrators for air travel use, as noted earlier in the discussion of oxygen concentrators.

Mechanical Ventilation

The current technology for noninvasive ventilation uses a face or nasal mask with a compressor that provides positive pressure which augments the patient's respiratory efforts. Although this has replaced earlier forms of noninvasive ventilation, it would be remiss not to mention these earlier forms. The first NIVS device was the rocking bed used for patients with polio, and about the same time the iron lung (negative pressure tank ventilator) was developed. The cuirass or "shell" ventilator was a more refined negative pressure ventilator, which could be fitted to the individual patient's chest wall and was portable. The purpose of these devices was to produce negative pressure to assist diaphragm movement. Although effective, the major drawbacks to these devices were their size and lack of patient acceptance.

Noninvasive Positive Pressure Ventilation

Continuous positive airway pressure ventilation (CPAP) and bi-level positive pressure ventilation (BiPAP) are the commonly used types of noninvasive positive-pressure ventilation (NPPV). CPAP maintains continuously positive airway pressure throughout the respiratory cycle and is most commonly used to treat patients with obstructive sleep apnea. The most effective setting (usually from 5 to 20 cm H_2O pressure) is determined during a sleep study. Because O_2 saturation is continuously measured at the same time, supplemental O_2 in addition to CPAP level can be titrated to maintain saturation at $\geq 90\%$. Newer forms of CPAP allow for a slow increase in the pressure (ramping), which helps some patients tolerate the support better. The most recent development allows for a pressure adjustment during exhalation (C-flex) so that the perception of increased airway pressure is not noticeable.

With other forms of respiratory insufficiency BiPAP provides more effective ventilatory support. BiPAP allows independent adjustment of the inspiratory and expiratory pressures that are delivered to the patient. Switching from inspiratory positive pressure (IPAP) to expiratory positive pressure (EPAP) is flow-triggered and time-limited. As with CPAP, BiPAP titration (with or without O_2) is best done in a sleep lab. Sometimes this is not possible, and empiric settings are chosen with IPAP ranging from 10 to 20 cm H_2O pressure and EPAP ranging from 5 to 15 cm H_2O pressure.

Most patients have some difficulty adjusting to NPPV, and home oxygen companies and other suppliers must troubleshoot. Physicians should select equipment suppliers that are "patient responsive" and eagerly assist patients. Some of the more common problems include mask intolerance, nasal congestion with dryness, nasal bridge redness with occasional ulceration, gastric insufflation, and air leaking through the mouth. Usually with different mask sizes and styles, careful adjustment of pressures, and the addition of humidification, patients can tolerate NPPV. Patients can use NPPV not only with sleep but for rest periods during the day. There is the occasional patient who prefers to have a tracheostomy and use BiPAP for assisted ventilation. It is appropriate to periodically (every 6-8 months) monitor nocturnal oxygen saturation at home to ensure that patients remain normoxemic during sleep.

Tracheostomy and Standard Positive Pressure Ventilation

While the use of chronic portable ventilators is becoming more common among younger patients, and especially those with spinal cord injury, it is uncommon for elderly patients to select this support. Most elderly patients who end up with a tracheostomy and chronic ventilator support have experienced one or more episodes of acute respiratory failure and have been unable to wean from standard mechanical ventilation after the last event. Some of these patients can be switched to nocturnal BiPAP through the tracheostomy, which is easier to manage in the home setting. When patients elect to discontinue ventilator support, adequate sedation and narcotics should be given. Air hunger, anxiety, and dyspnea can be eliminated with appropriate pharmacologic intervention (see Chapter 15).

Summary

In hypoxemic patients with COPD and other chronic lung diseases, long-term oxygen therapy improves survival and quality of life. The goal of therapy in LTOT is to maintain the partial pressure of oxygen at 55 mm Hg or greater, or the arterial oxygen saturation at 90% or above for 15-24 hours per day. This goal should be within reach for the vast majority of elderly patients with chronic pulmonary diseases. The challenges will be to continue improving respiratory care while reducing costs and to continue adding to the legacy of the pioneers in the field of LTOT.

Noninvasive ventilation is now delivered via a nasal or face mask. These have replaced the "iron lung" and "shell ventilator" of the past, which were unwieldy and inconvenient. CPAP and BiPAP are the most commonly used types of NPPV.

BIBLIOGRAPHY AND SUGGESTED READING

Hillberg RE, Johnson DC. Noninvasive ventilation. N Engl J Med. 1997;337:1746-52. *Review describing developments in noninvasive positive-pressure ventilation.*

Hoffman LA. Transtracheal oxygen therapy. Up to Date. February 15, 2002. *Concise review of the benefits and pitfalls of transtracheal oxygen therapy.*

Petty TL. Guide to Prescribing Home Oxygen. National Lung Health Education Program. http://www.nlhep.org. *Excellent, concise, overview of long-term oxygen therapy by a pioneer in the field.*

Petty TL. Supportive therapy in COPD. Chest. 1998;113:256S-262S. *Excellent discussion of supportive care for patients with COPD including oxygen therapy.*

Quinnell TG, Smith IE. Obstructive sleep apnea in the elderly: recognition and management considerations. Drugs Aging. 2004;21:307-22. *Outlines the use of continuous positive airway pressure in elderly patients with sleep apnea.*

Sutherland ER, Cherniack RM. Management of chronic obstructive pulmonary disease. N Engl J Med. 2004;350:2689-97. *Overview of treatment of COPD with extensive references.*

Tiep BL. Oxygen-conserving devices. Up to Date. July 30, 2002. *Excellent outline and review of oxygen conserving devices.*

Tiep BL, Carter R. Long-term supplemental oxygen therapy. Up to Date. January 16, 2004. *Well-organized and timely reference to long-term oxygen therapy.*

14 Progressive Respiratory Impairment

As aging occurs, there is a natural decline in man's cardiopulmonary performance, his reserve, and, eventually, his ability to sustain biological life. Numerous medical conditions affect and frequently accelerate the process. This chapter focuses on the most common causes of progressive respiratory insufficiency in the elderly, reviews appropriate diagnostic studies, and summarizes existing management options.

Etiology

Although there are numerous specific causes of progressive respiratory insufficiency, the two most common are congestive heart failure (CHF) and chronic obstructive lung disease (COPD). Rapid progression of symptoms and clinical deterioration occur when other secondary insults develop. These include acute myocardial ischemia, pneumonia, atelectasis, aspiration, acute blood loss, metabolic disorders, and sepsis. Specific therapies for these acute insults should be used appropriately. Some of the elderly have progressive respiratory insufficiency related to underlying malignancies and the associated chemotherapy and radiation treatment.

The causes of progressive respiratory insufficiency can be categorized in many ways. One practical approach outlines the causes as pulmonary, cardiac, neuromuscular, or related to sleep disorders or metabolic abnormalities (Table 14-1). It is not the purpose of this chapter to review each of the potential etiologies and their therapies in detail, but rather to discuss the end result: progressive respiratory insufficiency. In this discussion the assumption is made

Table 14-1 Causes of Progressive Respiratory Insufficiency in the Elderly

1. Obstructive lung disease

   - Emphysema & chronic bronchitis (COPD)
   - Bronchiectasis
   - Asthma

2. Restrictive lung disease

   - Idiopathic interstitial lung disease
   - Chronic aspiration pneumonitis
   - Surgical resection of lung tissue (pneumonectomy, lobectomy)
   - Sarcoidosis
   - Radiation pneumonitis

3. Cardiac disease

   - Coronary artery disease
   - Hypertensive cardiovascular heart disease
   - Valvular heart disease
   - Idiopathic cardiomyopathy

4. Musculoskeletal abnormalities

   - Kyphoscoliosis
   - Thoracoplasty

5. Neuromuscular disease

   - Post-polio syndrome
   - Amyotrophic lateral sclerosis
   - Myasthenia gravis
   - Phrenic nerve paralysis
   - Brain stem cerebrovascular accidents
   - Multiple sclerosis

6. Sleep and metabolic disorders

   - Obstructive sleep apnea syndrome
   - Central sleep apnea
   - Obesity hypoventilation syndrome
   - Hypothyroidism
   - Chronic electrolyte imbalance (e.g., hypokalemia, hypomagnesemia)

that the underlying cause has been identified and treated when possible, and the clinician is now left to manage the patient's chronic respiratory failure.

Clinical Presentation

The clinical presentation of progressive respiratory insufficiency (PRI) is variable and ranges from mild confusion to acute respiratory failure with hypoxemia and hypercapnia requiring intubation and mechanical ventilation. Those patients who are aware of progressive symptoms complain of increasing dyspnea on exertion, increased fatigue, weak muscles, orthopnea, paroxysmal nocturnal dyspnea, and eventually dyspnea at rest. At times it is a family member who notices a change in the patient's behavior and performance. Simple tasks such as personal care and verbal communication diminish. Environmental awareness and a desire to participate are no longer present. Earlier in the progression of disease, symptoms may be more specifically related to the underlying etiology, but dyspnea is the common theme. For example, the patient with severe COPD will also complain of chest tightness, mucus production, and panic attacks, while those with CHF note increased edema, exertional chest pain, and extreme fatigue. The physiologic abnormality in common to these patients is a reduced ability to deliver oxygen to the tissues (low oxygen saturation and reduced cardiac output) and/or an inability to remove carbon dioxide. When the patient becomes end-stage, combined cardio-respiratory failure frequently exists.

Diagnosis

The physical examination varies with the etiology of the respiratory insufficiency, and the astute physician quickly focuses on the important observations: general appearance (weight), mental status, bradycardia or tachycardia, hypertension or hypotension, crackles, rhonchi, wheezes, gallop, rhythm, murmurs, pulsatile liver, jugular venous distension, cyanosis, chest wall abnormalities, symmetrical chest wall expansion, diaphragmatic excursion, edema, clubbing, gait, muscle strength and tone, deep tendon reflex quality, fasciculations, and strength and quality of voice. The hallmark of severe chronic respiratory failure is pulmonary hypertension manifested by cor pulmonale with right-sided heart failure, increased pulmonic component of the second heart sound, tricuspid regurgitation, jugular venous distension, a pulsatile liver, and a right ventricular lift.

To define the severity of the respiratory insufficiency, specific tests of respiratory function are necessary. These include pulse oximetry, arterial blood gases (ABGs), spirometry, lung volumes, diffusing capacity, and measurement of negative inspiratory force. Helpful radiologic studies include chest x-ray, computed tomography, and diaphragmatic fluoroscopy. (For cardiac evaluation, see Chapter 10.) Sleep studies define the type and severity of sleep-disordered breathing.

Arterial Blood Gases and Pulse Oximetry

Pulse oximetry identifies patients with hypoxemia. Many patients with progressive respiratory insufficiency have chronic hypoxemia, and some continue to have hypoxemia despite supplemental oxygen. In patients with hypoxemia, the clinician must consider the classic physiologic abnormalities: 1) ventilation/perfusion mismatch; 2) right-to-left shunt; 3) hypoventilation; 4) diffusion abnormalities (a potential contributor to hypoxemia primarily during exercise); and 5) reduced inspired oxygen tension (altitude). Matching the physiologic principles to the clinical diagnosis defines the mechanism and cause of the respiratory insufficiency. When the resting O_2 saturation is normal, exercise oximetry should be performed. The 6-min walk is a simple means of measuring O_2 saturations with exercise and determining the distance a patient can cover. This test can be repeated to determine the patient's improvement or deterioration.

Although ABGs are invasive compared with pulse oximetry, they are extremely helpful in assessing acute and chronic respiratory insufficiency. In addition to providing information about O_2 saturation and partial pressure of oxygen (PaO_2), ABGs allow measurement of arterial pH and partial pressure of carbon dioxide ($PaCO_2$). When inadequate alveolar ventilation occurs, there is elevation in the $PaCO_2$. Acutely, the increased PCO_2 results in a fall in the arterial pH. A normal ABG has a pH of 7.40 and a PCO_2 of 38-42 mmHg (at sea level). With acute elevation of the PCO_2, the pH decreases by approximately 0.08 units for every 10 mm Hg increase in $PaCO_2$. Thus, a $PaCO_2$ of 50 mm Hg acutely results in a pH of approximately 7.32 (7.40-0.08). With time (several days), the patient retains serum bicarbonate to buffer the pH. Although the pH usually remains less than 7.40, the decrease is blunted by this renal compensation. With chronic elevation in $PaCO_2$, the pH decreases 0.03-0.04 units for every 10 mm Hg increase in $PaCO_2$. Thus, a chronically elevated $PaCO_2$ of 50 results in a pH of approximately 7.37 (7.40-0.03). With chronic CO_2 retention, the serum bicarbonate level increases 4 mEq/L for each 10 mm Hg increase in PCO_2. Thus, the typical finding in chronic respiratory failure with CO_2 retention is an increased $PaCO_2$ with a close-to-normal pH and an elevated serum bicarbonate. Some of the more common causes of chronically elevated $PaCO_2$ secondary to inadequate alveolar ventilation include 1) hypoventilation (COPD, obesity hypoventilation syndrome); 2) destruction of lung tissue (emphysema, end-stage ILD); 3) neuromuscular diseases (ALS, post-polio syndrome); and 4) restrictive disease from previous lung surgery or spine and chest wall abnormalities. Patients with primarily CHF rarely have isolated elevation in $PaCO_2$, and other etiologies must be considered.

Pulmonary Function Studies

Simple spirometry remains one of the most valuable tests available to document severity of illness and the likelihood of progressive respiratory insufficiency. The test is effort-dependent. It measures the forced vital capacity

(FVC) and the forced expiratory volume at 1 second (FEV_1). With COPD the FEV_1 is reduced; with most of the other causes of respiratory insufficiency (see Table 14-1), the FVC is abnormally low. When the FEV_1 and FVC fall below 30% of predicted, there is severe impairment and, if not already present, the development of chronic respiratory failure. In general, when the FVC falls below 1 L, patients will require supplemental oxygen, and some also require nocturnal noninvasive ventilation devices to assist their breathing.

When patients present with chronic respiratory insufficiency and the FVC and FEV_1 are adequate (>50% predicted), lung volumes to determine total lung capacity, residual volume, and functional residual capacity will better define the abnormality (restrictive [including neuromuscular disease] vs. obstructive).

The diffusing capacity (DLCO) measures the ability of carbon monoxide to transfer from alveolar gas to capillary blood. With advanced disease this value is usually low. Occasionally the DLCO is disproportionally reduced compared with other pulmonary function studies. When this occurs, patients frequently have much higher oxygen requirements than would be expected from other studies.

Negative Inspiratory Force

This is a simple yet helpful test to measure inspiratory effort against a closed pressure manometer. The patient inspires as deeply as possible and a negative pressure is generated. The maximal pressure most individuals can generate is approximately –100 cm H_2O. This is effort-dependent, and the patient must be able to have a tight seal around the mouthpiece. Values of less than –50 cm H_2O indicate decreased inspiratory effort, and when the NIF is less than –25 cm H_2O, significant respiratory impairment exists.

Radiologic Studies

Because radiologic studies define anatomic abnormalities and not physiological impairment, they are rarely helpful in diagnosing the presence of progressive respiratory insufficiency. They are, however, extremely helpful in determining the underlying cause. Chest x-rays remain useful in daily management and early diagnosis, but computed tomography is far superior for evaluating parenchymal, mediastinal, vascular, and pleural structures (see Chapter 9).

Diaphragmatic fluoroscopy is extremely helpful in assessing diaphragm function. The "sniff test" (in which the patient closes the mouth and sniffs through the nose) documents diaphragmatic paralysis by demonstrating paradoxical movement of the involved diaphragm (motion with the inspiratory sniff is cephalad instead of caudad). Normal diaphragmatic excursion is 5-6 cm. With paresis there is reduced movement but no paradoxical motion.

Sleep Studies

The availability of portable home units to provide continuous oxygen saturation readings has made physicians aware of the problem of nocturnal desaturation. Many of these patients do not have classic sleep apnea but demonstrate severe desaturations because of underlying cardiac, pulmonary, or neuromuscular disease. Prolonged episodes of nocturnal desaturation lead to pulmonary hypertension, cor pulmonale, and even daytime hypoxemia. When symptoms suggesting sleep apnea (either central or obstructive) are also present, a formal sleep study (polysomnogram) should be performed. All patients with progressive respiratory insufficiency should have a nocturnal oxygen saturation study and if hypoxemia exists, supplement oxygen should be provided to keep O_2 saturation at >90%.

Treatment

Patient Discussion

Compared with establishing the cause and severity of chronic respiratory insufficiency, outlining appropriate therapy is more difficult. As with any medical illness, patients want to be cured. They regret and often resent having a chronic illness, one that requires daily interventions, especially with chronic oxygen use. Patients must be taught that their conditions and situations are not hopeless. Although changes in lifestyle, daily activities, sleep patterns, nutrition, and exercise are necessary, with enthusiastic encouragement from physicians, family members, and friends, patients can successfully adapt. Common misconceptions among patients with progressive respiratory insufficiency include:

1. There are medications that can "cure" my condition.
2. I should limit oxygen use so I can get stronger.
3. If I use oxygen all the time, I will become "addicted."
4. If I "push" myself physically I can work through the problem.
5. Non-traditional therapies can "cure" my illness.

The current treatments for PRI—medications, oxygen therapy, exercise, dietary supplements, and other therapies (e.g., yoga, acupuncture, support groups)—while they do not "cure" the condition, do improve quality of life and exercise tolerance, reduce despair, and offer hope. Because chronic respiratory insufficiency cannot be cured, patients must be educated and encouraged that their major goals are to prevent continued deterioration and focus on improved quality of life.

Most patients with progressive respiratory insufficiency want insight into "The Big Picture," but others may not, so the compassionate physician should ask specifically, "What do you want to know about your condition?" Responses will vary from "everything" to "just tell me when I'm going to die." The key is to open a dialogue so continued compassionate, honest, and encouraging discussions take place. It is absolutely impossible to adequately care for these patients without addressing end-of-life issues (see Chapter 15).

General Therapeutic Concepts

In patients with progressive respiratory insufficiency the following should be addressed:

1. Is drug therapy for the underlying disease optimal?
2. Is the patient's oxygen saturation >90% (rest, exercise, and sleep)?
3. Is the patient on any drugs that could make the condition worse?
4. Are any acute factors or illnesses causing deterioration?

For a variety of reasons, many patients resist using supplemental oxygen. Physicians must emphasize that the single most important therapy for patients who are hypoxemic (O_2 sat <88%, PaO_2 <55 mm Hg) is the use of supplemental oxygen.

If the patient remains symptomatic and physical findings and laboratory studies indicate progressive respiratory insufficiency, some form of assisted mechanical ventilatory support should be considered (see Chapter 13). For many patients, this represents a key crossroad. The two extremes in therapy range from "hospice with comfort-care measures only" to a tracheostomy with 24-hour ventilator support. Fortunately, there are therapeutic measures between the extremes.

Pharmacological Agents to Aid Comfort

An important concept in managing patients with progressive respiratory insufficiency should be emphasized. Even when patients are requesting a full resuscitation status, patient comfort with relief of dyspnea and pain is the primary goal. When specific drugs used to treat chronic cardio-respiratory insufficiency fail, narcotics, anti-anxiety agents, and sleeping aids should be offered. There is a general misconception that use of these agents is contraindicated in patients with progressive respiratory insufficiency because of accelerating respiratory failure. Starting with lower doses of narcotics (e.g., 5-10 mg of oxycodone or hydrocodone) every 4-6 hours is well tolerated. In some cases, the longer-acting oxycodone (OxyContin) may be appropriate in doses ranging from 10 to 80 mg every 12 hours. The goal is reduction of symptoms without over-sedation. Lorazepam (Ativan) effectively relieves anxiety. The usual starting dose is 0.5-1 mg every 6-8 hours. Because anxiety and hyperventilation produce increased respiratory distress, they should be treated and prevented. Many patients complain of poor-quality sleep, sometimes because they cannot tolerate noninvasive positive pressure ventilation. The periodic use of zolpidem (Ambien) 5-10 mg at bedtime is well tolerated in most patients. In patients with sleep-disordered breathing and NPPV, the addition of sleeping aids may improve quality of sleep.

The Key Role of the Managing Physician

The importance of healing the whole and not the parts is insisted on.

Sir William Osler

In elderly patients, the psychological impact of inexorable disease with attendant impaired quality of life requires the mature guidance and management of the caring physician. Compassionate care requires understanding of the patient's medical and psychosocial problems intertwined with an abundance of empathy. Just talking with patients in the office, hospital, nursing home, or by telephone is extremely helpful. Encouraging the patients to capitalize on good days and minimize the impact of bad days is an important strategy. Maintaining a hopeful attitude based upon reasoned optimism and unconditional commitment to continued care keeps most patients and their families at a high level of comfort and peace. Focusing on the spiritual aspects of aging and the dying process, and relating them to illness is often salutary. Helping the patient achieve spiritual tranquility salves the anxiety and uncertainty about the future and allows patients to participate in an enjoyable life. Avoiding the pain and suffering that may accompany death is a key strategy that must be understood by physician, patient, and family alike. There is no question that the complete physician understands the profound implications of the process of managing patients as they approach life's promised end.

> . . . and thus this man died leaving his death for an example of noble courage
> and of moral virtue.
>
> 2 Maccabees 6:31

Summary

In the absence of sudden death, progressive respiratory insufficiency occurs in most patients with COPD, ILD, CHF, and neuromuscular disease. With aggressive treatment of the underlying disorders and with the use of supplemental oxygen therapy, many patients maintain a good quality of life. Regular exercise, support groups, frequent outings, and spiritual enrichment all contribute to this quality. As the work of breathing increases, the addition of noninvasive positive pressure ventilation brings relief and helps to treat progressive respiratory insufficiency. Eventually the addition of narcotics, anxiolytics, and sleeping aids is necessary. Remember that, although a cure for progressive respiratory insufficiency is not possible, the goal of therapy is improved quality of life.

BIBLIOGRAPHY AND SUGGESTED READING

Adams FV. Healing through empathy. Lincoln, NE: iUniverse Inc; 2004. *Brief monograph based on seven patients with illnesses ranging from complex to life-threatening.*

Fries JF. Aging, natural death, and the compression of morbidity. N Engl J Med. 1980;303:130-5. *Comprehensive review about strategies to reduce morbidity in aging patients who ultimately face death.*

Petty TL. Managing death and other difficult situations. In: Petty TL. Intensive and Rehabilitative Respiratory Care, 3rd ed. Philadelphia: Lea & Febiger; 1982. *Chapter on death management.*

Vig EK, Pearlman RA. Good and bad dying from the perspective of terminally ill men. Arch Intern Med. 2004;164:977-81. *Provides patient views on quality of life while facing death.*

15 End-of-Life Matters

The days of our lives shall be three score and ten years, and if, by strength, they may be four score years . . . and then the spirit takes wings and flies away.

PSALMS 90:10

This chapter discusses many of the issues of end-of-life care and why it is so often mishandled. It is written from the perspective of both practicing pulmonologists and individuals who have practiced critical care medicine and ongoing care, including terminal care, for more than four decades.

In its medical context, life effectively ends when there is no meaningful interaction between patient, family, and environment, and after it is certain that basic mental functions will not return. It is not difficult to know when cognitive life has ended. When a persistent vegetative state in nontraumatic hypoxic head injury exists after 3 months, the probability of good recovery is only 1%. If that state exists for more than 6 months, the probability is zero. Examples of recovery from longstanding unconsciousness all have medical explanations. They are not relevant to the highly publicized cases of "clinically dead" patients such as Karen Ann Quinlan, Paul Brophy, Nancy Cruzan, and, most recently, Terri Schiavo.

Terri Schiavo, aged 26, suffered severe hypoxemia following a collapse in her apartment in February 1990. She had no living will or durable power of attorney. Approximately 4 months after her collapse, she was judged by a Florida court to be incompetent. Her husband, Michael Schiavo, was appointed her legal guardian without objection from her parents, the Schindlers. At first, Mrs Schiavo was supported by a percutaneous endoscopic gastrostomy (PEG) tube for nutrition. By late 1990, she was determined to be in a persistent vegetative state and her husband requested her feeding tube be removed. This action was vigorously opposed the Schindlers, who sought legal redress with the intention of having the feeding tube reinstated.

Many legal actions followed, including the passage of Florida legislation known as "Terri's Law" (allowing Governor Jeb Bush to order reinsertion of her feeding tube). Michael Schiavo challenged this legislation; the case was eventually brought before the Florida Supreme Court. This allowed a judge to hear the husband's testimony and that of three witnesses who testified to Terri's statements that "she would not want to live like that." This testimony convinced the judge that there was "clear and convincing evidence" that the PEG tube should be removed. After Terri's Law was overturned and the PEG tube removed, further courthouse testimony and appeals followed, actions which culminated in a special session of Congress called by President George W. Bush, which passed legislation that in effect called for the reinsertion of the feeding tube. The U.S. Supreme Court on appeal upheld the Florida Supreme Court ruling and the PEG tube was again removed. Terri Schiavo died in March 2005, more than 15 years after her collapse. At autopsy, her brain weighed only 615 g, about one-half of normal brain weight, and extensive cortical damage consistent with hypoxic-ischemic brain damage was found.

Although this case remains controversial, many jurists and physicians have argued that the Supreme Court decision was "an example of good standards and processes in medicine, law, and ethics" (Perry et al 2005). The central focus of the Schiavo case was patient autonomy and surrogate decision making, and it embodied the principle that self-determination is a fundamental right guaranteed by the Constitution. An important lesson should be learned from this controversy: the necessity of an unambiguous advance directive prepared in the event of catastrophic accident or illness.

Preparing for End of Life

Man is the only animal who knows he is mortal. "Nobody ever got off this planet alive" is a quote from Woody Allen. He also said, "I don't mind dying; I just don't want to be there when it happens."

In our discussions about end-of-life matters with patients and their families, however, we do not recommend such a lighthearted approach. Dying is a serious matter that is the natural end of living. We encourage our patients to understand that we will postpone death as long as is reasonable and possible; we also must be honest and forthright.

All patients should have discussions with their doctors and families, preferably at a time when they are still healthy, about what is commonly called "end-of-life decisions." These discussions are important even if death itself is far in the future, and they should be repeated periodically. This is a good rehearsal for the time when death is near. We suggest the term "decisions at the time of transition." This has spiritual connotations that can be individually interpreted. Having a clear understanding about what the patient wants done when facing a catastrophic situation, such as a persistent vegetative state, is of key importance. Everyone should have well documented personal wishes in the form of a Living Will or a durable medical Power of Attorney. These two documents provide for surrogate decision making in times of crisis. They do not necessarily require a lawyer.

The medical principles involved at end of life are not complex. The patient expects and is entitled to the best life-support care as long as meaningful recovery is possible. Beneficence is part of the tradition of medicine, as cited in the Hippocratic Oath: ". . .I will come for the benefit of the sick." The Florence Nightingale pledge includes the phrase: ". . . and devote myself to the welfare of those committed to my care." The autonomy of the individual is guaranteed by fundamental principles, including the Constitution, which guarantees the right to privacy, and Common Law, which determines the right to bodily self-determination.

Informed consent is another fundamental principle. In medicine, informed consent means truth telling about any and all possibilities that may occur during medical care. Informed consent is implicit in the Living Will and Power of Attorney. The patient consents to be treated or not, and the patient or a surrogate can demand that life support be withdrawn. The President's Commission has clearly stated that there is no moral, ethical, or legal difference between withholding treatment and withdrawing it in hopeless situations.

Finally, the principle of the patient's best interests is intertwined in all of the above. Is it sound medical care to continue life support for a patient in a persistent vegetative state with a feeding tube or a respirator?

The day will come when all must face their death. Very few of us want to die. Most of us are frightened by the imminence of death. Most patients want to know: How will it happen? Will I suffer? Will I suffocate? Will I have uncontrollable anxiety? Will I writhe in pain? Is it possible to face death with some control over these fears?

A frequent question asked of physicians treating patients with severe COPD, interstitial lung disease, or lung cancer is "How long do I have to live?" The honest response is "I don't know." Two patients with COPD may have identical seriousness of illness medically, yet one lives several months, even years longer than the other. It is difficult to explain why and how some patients can live, in some cases, far beyond what is expected.

All patients should be told that there are many medications that can control pain and anxiety. Patients do not need to have "everything done" to provide for their comfort and quality of life. Ventilation may not be needed to stop the feeling of suffocation that accompanies a severe attack of COPD. Appropriate use of narcotics, particularly morphine and sedatives, can control shortness of breath and pain. The dying body prepares for death by gradually shutting down organ system functions, such as the kidneys and digestive tract. This does *not* cause hunger or thirst. It brings nature's relief. It is important for the patient and all involved in his or her care to resolve that death is not an enemy. Patients fear loneliness, pain, and other suffering, but not death itself. Death is a natural process, unless interference unnaturally extends the time to death and prevents its spiritual meaning.

For patients with severe COPD, there may come a time when quality of life is so poor, pain so severe, and breathlessness so intolerable that life seems to have no purpose. At this point, the patient's emotional and physical comfort must come first. The goal is no longer to "tough-it-out" but to find peace and comfort within one's self, with family, and with friends. This acceptance and the use of comfort measures do not mean death is immediate; they mean that the patient has taken control. Neither COPD nor any other disease should dominate the patient's daily life.

For many patients, when the decision not to continue living has been reached, support from home care agencies may be welcome or they may choose to spend their final days in a hospice. Both home care and hospice workers provide compassionate and understanding physical, emotional, and spiritual support.

The Five Wishes Program

The Five Wishes Program: Aging with Dignity (The Robert Wood Johnson Foundation, Princeton, New Jersey) has been widely promoted and acclaimed. The Five Wishes Program embodies and clarifies or expands on the advance directive that can be used to guide surrogate decision making.

Because there are many aspects of life that are out of patients' control, especially when serious illness is present, the Five Wishes booklet was created as an easy-to-complete form that allows the patient to say exactly what he or she wants. The beauty of the document is its simplicity combined with sensitivity and specificity. It was written with the help of the American Bar Association's Commission on the Legal Problems of the Elderly and the nation's leading experts on end-of-life care. Five Wishes is for anyone 18 or older. Because it works so well, lawyers, doctors, hospitals, hospices, religious organizations, employers, and retiree groups are handing out this document.

Wish 1: My wish for the person I want to make health care decisions for me when I can't make them for myself

This section of the Program tells how to obtain a durable medical Power of Attorney. It contains a full discussion of whom the patient should select as his or her surrogate decision maker and the specific obligations the patient should require of that person.

Wish 2: My wish for the kind of medical treatment I want or don't want

This wish is equivalent to a combination of the Living Will and the Advance Resuscitation Directive. It explains what "Do Not Resuscitate" (DNR) means in simple but explicit lay terms. Specifics of what the patient wants done in the following settings are listed:

1. Close to death
2. In a coma and not expected to wake up or recover
3. Permanent and severe brain damage and not expected to recover

Wish 3: My wish for how comfortable I want to be

This section of the Program covers pain medication, hands-on care such as bathing or massages, comforting music, and personal spiritual needs.

Wish 4: My wish for how I want people to treat me

Discussed in this section are personal visitation, attitudes the patient wants conveyed at the bedside, the desire for visitor prayer and spiritual support, and a clarification of where the patient wants to die (e.g., home, hospice).

Wish 5: My wish for what I want my loved ones to know

A wonderful selection of personal requests is provided. There may be statements about how much someone is loved, a request for forgiveness, a request for family and friends to make peace and bond during the patient's dying process, and a specific request for burial or cremation.

Summary

Advance directives clarify what patients want regarding medical care at end of life. Their purpose is to make certain each individual's desires and wishes are followed. Advance directives do not remove hope or the desire for life; they *give* patients control, freedom, comfort, and peace.

The tragedy of life is not that it ends so soon, but that we wait so long to begin it.
W. M. LEWIS

BIBLIOGRAPHY AND SUGGESTED READING

Hanson LC, Ersek M. Meeting palliative care needs in post-acute care settings: "to help them live until they die". JAMA. 2006;295:681-6. *Patient-based discussion on palliative care practices and principles for a patient who was dying of metastatic melanoma with pulmonary and CNS involvement.*

Hastings Center. Guideline on the Termination of Life-Sustaining Treatment and the Care of the Dying. Bloomington: Indiana University Press; 1987. *Commonly referenced historical guideline.*

Mower WR, Baraff LJ. Advance directives: effect of type of directive on physicians' therapeutic decisions. Arch Intern Med. 1993;153:375-81. *Analysis of the impact of end-of-life wishes and physician decisions.*

Perry JE, Churchill LR, Kirshner HS. The Terri Schiavo Case: legal, ethical, and medical perspectives. Ann Intern Med. 2005;143:744-8. *Review of the Terri Schiavo case. Stresses the importance of all patients having an advance directive, particularly when young and in good health.*

Snyder L, Leffler C, for the Ethics and Human Rights Committee, American College of Physicians. Ethics Manual, 5th ed. Ann Intern Med. 2005;142:561-83. *Contains a valuable section on care of patients near the end of life. The manual is also available from ACP in booklet form.*

Teno J, Lynn J, Wenger N, et al. Advance directives for seriously ill hospitalized patients: effectiveness with the patient self-determination act and the SUPPORT intervention. SUPPORT Investigators. Study to Understand Prognoses and Preferences for Outcomes and Risks of Treatment. J Am Geriatr Soc. 1997;45:500-7. *Commonly quoted reference.*

Index

A

CORE COLLECTION 2007